Beyond Domestication

Empowering Your
Physical, Mental, Emotional
& Spiritual Well-Being
Through Rewilding

George Knight

Hatherleigh Press is committed to preserving and protecting
the natural resources of the earth. Environmentally
responsible and sustainable practices are embraced
within the company's mission statement.

Visit us at www.hatherleighpress.com.

BEYOND DOMESTICATION

Library of Congress Cataloging-in-Publication
Data is available upon request.
ISBN: 978-1-57826-988-4

Cover Design by Ali Al Amine
Interior Design by Carolyn Kasper

Printed in the United States
10 9 8 7 6 5 4 3 2 1

CONTENTS

THE SEVEN PRACTICES FOR WELL-BEING

WE WERE ONCE wild.

When the first humans started walking the Earth, we were just another part of the circle of life, another part of the food chain. Evolving over millions of years, our ancient ancestors performed a vital role in the sustainability of our planet. Moving through different environments, they foraged local foods, hunted local animals, harvested dead wood for fire and lived in harmony with their environment.

For millions of years, they spread throughout the world, developing new skills along the way that made us capable of surviving in ever harsher environments.

But these new skills came at a price. As our descendants continued to spread through the new world, they developed a new form of intelligence. An intelligence that they used to interfere with the natural order on Earth.

They sacrificed a rich and varied wild diet for an industry propped up by animal suffering and nutrition-less plants.

Their water, which used to flow uninterrupted from the highest mountains to the sea, they dammed and stored, impacting countless other species (including humans).

The air they breathe became polluted as a side-effect of economic growth, as they burnt thousands of tons of fossil fuels that were previously trapped under the surface of the Earth for hundreds of millions of years.

They even said goodbye to the sun as they retreated indoors. Life under the sky became a life under a ceiling.

As for the people that inhabit this new Earth, they gave up movement for sedentarism. Mindfulness became distraction, and sleep became a chore dictated by numbers ticking on a clock.

We are now facing the harshest environment humans have ever faced. Increasing numbers of people are eating ultra-processed food. We are witnessing clean water shortages, dangerous levels of air pollution and a concerning increase in the number of people experiencing poor mental health.

We have forgotten about the land we evolved in sustainably for millions of years for this man-made dystopia, rejecting all that is natural for all that is unnatural.

As new generations are born, they take up the previous mantle, assuming it to be correct, blindly and boldly forging deeper down this path.

But where did this all start?

At what point did humans gain the power to destabilize our world?

When we got the power, why did we use it against the planet that has given us everything?

This book is the story of how my journey towards remission for Crohn's disease and my experience of bunions uncovered the greater need for humans and the planet to rewild.

You will quickly see that Crohn's and toes were just catalysts and that my rewilding journey quickly became about more than just my physical health.

To guide us on this rewilding journey, we will spend time with each of the Seven Practices for Well-being:

- Food
- Water
- Air
- Sunlight
- Movement
- Mindfulness
- Sleep

The Seven Practices are a product of the rewilding journey that my wife and co-founder at Beyond Domestication, Amber-Rose, and I have been on since 2016.

The book will be split into nine chapters, with the first chapter introducing rewilding for well-being. We will then explore each of the Seven Practices over the following seven chapters. We will look at how each practice plays a role in the health and well-being of humans and the planet's health.

The last chapter will conclude what we have looked at and explore how we can continue our Seven Practices rewilding journey.

This book will give you a deeper insight into the impact that Food, Water, Air, Sunlight, Movement, Mindfulness and Sleep have on health and well-being. Each chapter will challenge and hopefully energize you to kickstart your well-being journey by reconnecting to nature.

At the end of each chapter, you will find a summary of recommendations for you to try and practice in your life.

This book is not medical advice, and the Seven Practices are not a substitution for modern healthcare. If you are currently seeing a doctor or on medication, let that give you a platform for wellness and speak to a healthcare professional if you have any questions about how the Seven Practices can help you in your journey. Each recommendation in this book must be considered in the context of your health and well-being.

I will consider this book a success if you have taken away the importance of having a positive relationship with the Seven Practices upon reading it. That relationship will be different for everybody; only you can take this journey.

INTRODUCTION
WHY REWILD?

I **WAS FIRST DRAWN** to learn about rewilding through our relationship to food and the benefits it can have on health.

I was diagnosed with Crohn's disease before my 10th birthday. I spent most of my childhood and young adulthood catering, in some way, to the demands that an incurable illness supposedly brings.

As someone who suffered from Crohn's disease, I always paid close attention to my food. But, despite that interest, throughout my childhood, I still ate a typical western diet. I just did not know better.

I was fortunate to be in this position, and my parents always did their best to provide high-quality meals with various plants and animals. But I was still eating only domesticated animals and plants alongside the typical processed, sugary treats and drinks marketed so well to us.

Mine and Amber's research into a cleaner, healthier, more sustainable way of eating was our gateway into the rewilding community. Changing both of our diets and seeing the benefits that it brought physically and mentally was enough to get us both hooked on the path of rewilding.

From there, my journey took me to movement, while Amber's journey took her to mindfulness. My movement journey saw me heal the bunions on my feet, whilst my feet grew (and spread) from a size seven to nine over three years, just from moving better and wearing different footwear.

Amber's journey with mindfulness focused on her mental health and her evolution from a career as a photographer to a leader in the HR profession. She used the mindfulness practice to reflect honestly on her past and plan successfully for the future.

We kept returning to the Practices as we continued rewilding our well-being. From Food, we explored our relationship with the elements: the Water we drink, the Air we breathe, and our exposure to Sunlight. Our journey with Sleep came last, bringing us to the Seven Practices for Well-being we use today.

We were forging a new pathway to well-being for ourselves, and we needed to let others know. Beyond Domestication was born to share that story, creating a healthier, more sustainable path for us, our family, friends, and the wider community.

The good news is that in July 2021, I got a letter from my doctor with test results saying: "No active Crohn's." After 21 years, I had achieved a major breakthrough. Incorporating and following the Seven Practices, along with the support of the NHS, gave me the platform of health to achieve remission. Something I never thought was possible to fight for.

Remission is a two-way street, and I will always be thankful for the support of the NHS in allowing me to feel well while on my journey. Auto-immune diseases like Crohn's can be finicky beasts, as some readers will know, and it may be naïve to think this is the end of my health story. With the Seven Practices to guide me, I will continue keeping a close eye on my health as I support myself through my lifestyle choices.

To continue our journey in this book, let us look backwards at the time when humans chose another path.

The Great Forgetting

Around 11,000 years ago, in Göbekli Tepe, now an archaeological site located in Turkey, people began to domesticate plants and animals. Historical analysis of the site reveals it as the one of the oldest known records of agriculture.[1]

Since then, this type of food production has dominated the planet, with only a few million inhabitants not living within the human society governed by this form of agriculture.

Historians have named this change in approach to food production and society the agricultural revolution, and since its invention, this way of providing food has dominated almost every other method.

Other forms of agriculture were practiced at a much smaller scale by specific indigenous groups years before that fateful event in Göbekli Tepe, but without the overarching consequences that our form of agriculture has led to.

It is important to note now that farming is not the enemy. Farming may have been a natural step for humans as Göbekli Tepe was not the only site where farming began to occur. Maybe this was a step we were always destined to take as a species, and this book will look at the ways to be well, healthy and happy humans alongside agriculture.

---

1   Symmes, 2010

Over the last 11,000 years, humans have experienced a great forgetting of many practices that our ancestors had been utilizing for over 300,000 years. As agriculture continued to grow and proliferate, many unique indigenous societies and their respective lifestyles and practices were lost.

There is much more to be said about this critical stage in humanity's development, but you do not need to know more to rewild your well-being! If you are interested, I recommend the wonderful books Sapiens by Yuval Noah Harari and Wild New World by Dan Flores.

This taming of our world has led to the global society that most people form a part of today. Right now, most humans are part of a massive, dynamic, global network of countries, corporations and communities, with only a small few hunter-gatherer tribes living outside of that bubble.

Most of "us" (if you are reading this book, I strongly suspect you to be part of this us) are all living, eating and breathing within the same society. There are cultural differences that come with living in different places. However, despite these cultural differences, most of us still live and work in the same society.

So, what lessons did we lose and do they even matter?

Our society has tamed our planet into supporting an incredibly high number of humans, infant mortality keeps getting lower, life expectancy mostly keeps increasing, and we have developed the technology to make it out of our atmosphere and into the solar system.

However, we are not perfect. The planet is wracked with climate emergencies. People are still starving despite the abundance of food, the top 1 percent of earners are getting disproportionately wealthier and mental health is now the leading cause of illness worldwide.

What if we take the time to pause and reflect whilst we still can?

We must remember that our ancestors have been evolving alongside nature for 300,000 years. We owe it to the future of humanity to ensure that the relationship this generation and the next build with nature allows both humans and the planet to thrive.

There is no going backwards. Not for now, at least, as we will find out now with this story about one of our many extinct species, the auroch.

Story of the Auroch

In 2015, a farm in Cornwall, England, had to thin a herd of their cattle because they were too aggressive. These unique cows, named Heck cattle after brothers Lutz and Heinz Heck, were the descendants of an experiment from the middle of the 20th century.

Heck cattle were the outcome of a 1930s experiment to bring back the auroch—the wild progenitor of the domesticated cow. Lutz and Heinz Heck believed that selectively breeding existing cattle species for distinctive features (horn shape, coloration and aggressive behavior) could revert these domesticated cattle's genetic line to the wild auroch.

If you have not heard of the auroch before, you may have seen a drawing of one. Images of aurochs are included among the cave paintings drawn by indigenous artists at the Chalet cave in France, estimated to have been completed 15,000 years ago.

The auroch once roamed free across much of Eurasia and North Africa, playing a keystone role in the ecosystems it was a part of. Similar to the role of bison in North America (and now Europe).

When an animal has a keystone role in its ecosystem, many other species rely on its presence to survive. One of the challenges faced by ecosystems worldwide is the loss of keystone species. In the water chapter, we will discuss another keystone species, the beaver.

When the last known auroch was killed in the forests of Poland in the early 1600s, we were left with just the cow, the version of the auroch domesticated by humans many thousands of years earlier.

Like how we domesticated the grey wolf into a dog, we created the docile cow from the dangerous auroch. But unlike the wolf, the auroch was killed off.

However, scientists Luts and Heinz Heck believed they could rewild the cow through radical breeding practices. They aimed to undo the thousands of years of domestication submitted to the species by selectively breeding specific characteristics.

Lutz Heck travelled Europe selecting the most suitably horned and aggressive animals before returning to unite them into a single breeding stock.

At the time, the study was considered a success as they had created an animal with a mean temperament and the hardiness to survive in the wild. But, this research took place before the discovery of DNA, so Lutz and Heinz could never objectively validate their experiment's success.

Future studies of the descendants of Lutz and Heinz's Heck cattle showed that their experiment had not been a complete success. They were a tough breed but still lacked certain genes and distinct characteristics of the auroch.

The outcome of this experiment could be an early sign for the future of native biodiversity on Earth that evolution is a linear journey and that the species we have already lost due to the actions of our society might be just that—lost.

All is not lost, though, as analysis into the domestication of keystone species like the auroch has continued, with alternative studies producing more substantial results than Lutz and Heinz Heck were capable of.

Programs like the Tauros Programme demonstrate how continuing selective breeding of hardy cattle can bring some superficial resemblance to the now-extinct aurochs.[2] These hardy cattle are now being used throughout Europe in rewilding conservation programs.

This could be the beginning of a new future for all life on Earth that has, through contact with Homo sapiens, become domesticated in one way or another.

One day, pigs, sheep, dogs, cats, chickens, donkeys, camels, horses and all the other domesticated animals may once again be seen in adequate numbers in their vital roles, supporting the ecosystems of Earth.

Domestication is not just a problem for animals. We have also overseen the domestication of countless plants, such as lettuce, barley, rice, peanuts, grapes, bananas, and apples. Like our wild animals, each wild plant on our planet also evolved for a specific purpose (more on this in the Food chapter).

Can we afford to keep taking from Mother Nature without any plan of returning what she created?

---

2   Tauros | Rewilding Europe, n.d.

Now is the time to discover a path *beyond* domestication, where we balance the needs of our planet against the needs of our society.

Domestication of Humanity

Our journey with domestication is not just important for the future of our planet and the many species it hosts but also for the future of humans.

As I write this, I sit comfortably on a yoga mat in my one-bed flat in Camden Town, London. I have an extractor fan system that cleans the air in the flat, double-glazed windows that keep the elements out, and a lightning-fast internet connection that I can use to order anything I could ever imagine.

I am surrounded by modern gadgets and gizmos designed to make my life easier. If you compare this to the life our ancestors lived for 95 percent of the last 300,000 years, the differences could not be more striking.

Our lifestyles have been tamed. Our lack of physical trials and time in nature alongside an increase in comforts has gradually led, over time, to the domestication of the modern human.

If you say our hunter-gatherer ancestors are like the wild grey wolves we see today, then we have become the pug. One big difference, we are failing to recognize our domestication.

Science correctly categorizes the grey wolf and its domesticated descendants as *Canis lupus* and *Canis domesticus*, respectively. Should we be doing the same thing for us?

If we are no longer the wild, resilient *Homo sapien*, have we become the tame *Homo domesticus*, just like our furry friends did?

This argument was taken a step further when researchers in Spain compared the genes of modern humans to those of domesticated animals to try and establish if we are presenting genes that would typically be associated with domestication.

When they compared the genes of the domesticated dog and current humans against the genes of a wolf and a neanderthal, they found that both the dog's and human's genes had altered in a similar pattern, suggesting domestication has occurred equally in both the dog and us.[3]

Now, this is just one study. But if we believe in Darwinism, that we are constantly evolving as a response to our environment, isn't it possible that human domestication is true?

Are we slowly going down a rabbit hole towards a world where our health and diversity are at risk?

Or is there still time to move towards a wild world of respect and resilience amongst all species?

There can be both good and bad outcomes along this genetic journey that we find ourselves walking on. The first step is for humans to stop and recognize that we are on this journey in the first place.

Domestication is "the process of taming an animal or cultivating a plant," and taming something is "to make it less powerful and easier to control." We knew what we were doing when we domesticated all of our livestock by selecting and breeding for preferable characteristics, but we are only just realizing the impact that this has.

Right now, there are only an estimated 10 million people still living a hunter-gatherer lifestyle. We have already experienced

---

3   Theofanopoulou et al., 2018

one great forgetting. What will we lose if one day there are no human communities left with the space or environment to live sustainably off the land outside of the systems our society has created? We still have time to recognize our domestication and support these communities still living sustainably off the land.

One of the most significant changes to our body during domestication is the size of our brains. Compared to our wild ancestors who lived only 10,000–20,000 years ago, our brains have shrunk in comparison by 10–15 percent.

We do not yet know how much of an impact this has had on our cognitive abilities. Still, it is strange to think that our brains have gotten smaller as we created this technological world using only human imagination and science.

Two leading theories are that as society developed and the first towns and villages were built, it became possible for people to be more sedentary. This reduction in movement caused brain sizes to shrink.

Or that as we continued to work in bigger and bigger groups of people, we experienced a natural selection that favored humans capable of working well with their fellow humans, compared to natural selection, which typically favored more physical capabilities.[4]

Domestication came at us fast because that is what it does. Domestication does not slowly take place over thousands of years like evolution. It occurs quickly, sometimes taking only a few generations.

We know this because we only recently domesticated the silver fox. Still a wild animal in many parts of the world, the silver

---

4   Stringer, 2014

fox was chosen as the subject of a domestication experiment in Russia.

In 1959, Russian geneticist Lyudmila Trut began to selectively breed docile and friendly foxes in the opposite approach to Lutz and Heinz Heck and their angry cattle program.

After only ten years, in 1969, they started to see radical changes in the mood, fur color and ear shape, among other characteristics of the fox. These changes mirror the similar pattern that dogs have gone through in their adaption from wolves.[5]

Despite evolution moving slowly over thousands of years, domestication can occur in just a few generations. Now think about how far back you would have to look in your family tree to find your last indigenous ancestor.

Many of us have no clue how far down the domestication tunnel our genes have walked, and it is likely significantly more than a few generations have passed since your last wild ancestor was alive.

Domestication is a real threat to humans, and we are all responsible for giving our mind and body the wild feedback it needs to thrive.

It must be said that certain aspects of domestication have provided benefits to our society. But we risk destabilizing the balance upon which our global ecosystem relies when we do irresponsible things like wipe out the wild progenitor of a species.

Despite the downsides to domestication, the way humanity has spread throughout the globe has been highly successful. This more cooperative but less physical society of humans has dominated every other species into submission and is learning

5   Dugatkin and Trut, 2017

more and more each day about how to shape the world to do its bidding.

Mental Health

One of the biggest changes to daily life in the last few decades is the advancement of the digital world. As our relationship with digital technology grows, we have seen a significant increase in people suffering from poor mental health. Physical injuries suffered in fields and industrial factories used to be the main concern. Now, we have the psychological impact of a digital life disconnected from nature.

When we packed up our bags and left the forest for our artificial towns and cities, our mental health was impacted alongside our physical health. Studies have shown that when compared to their wild ancestors, domesticated animals present more anxious behavior, take fewer risks, and explore less.[6]

Sound familiar?

We already know that we share similarities with the domesticated dog. Is it likely that humans are also experiencing a similar behavior change?

Anxiety, alongside other forms of mental health, is now the leading cause of ill health and disability worldwide. The British charity Mind says that one-in-four people will experience poor mental health at some point.[7]

Whether this is due to the environments we live in, the bombardment of social media or something else entirely, we

---

6   Kaiser, Hennessy and Sachser, 2015

7   How common are mental health problems?, 2020

face a different kind of global pandemic that continues spiraling downwards each year, leaving nobody unaffected.

Beyond Domestication

To uncover the answers to my well-being. I looked first at our ancestors and considered how I could mimic their experiences within my life, despite our lifestyles taking place in vastly different environments.

People around the globe are choosing to connect to nature in the few areas of wilderness that still exist. Everywhere we look, people are trying to rewild themselves, rediscovering the wisdom of the past and integrating these skills into their modern lifestyle.

One of the wilder people in our society is Lynx Vilden. Lynx is one of the world's leading practitioners of primitive skills and has been teaching stone age practices for decades. Her tribe of dedicated and like-minded individuals run two-month immersions where they mimic the life of a stone-age tribe, leaving the material world behind and using only what has been made personally from the land. No metals, no glass, no plastics and no cloth.

These immersions provide a unique opportunity to live as our ancestors did, but I am not suggesting that we all pack up and pursue the same lifestyle. We have come too far as a society to throw away all that progress now. But Lynx and her tribe show that physically and mentally, humans *can* still operate in our pre-domesticated lifestyle.

On the other end of the spectrum is the life that many humans are now leading. A life where we fail to get the fundamentals of our well-being right. And right now, the well-being fundamental for many humans is to spend more time in nature.

Science supports the argument that nature is good for our well-being. When 38 healthy city-dwellers went for a 90-minute walk through a natural environment, they reported lower levels of rumination (negative thoughts). Their brain scans showed reduced activity in the area linked to sadness, withdrawal and grumpiness. The results also showed that time in nature increased positive thoughts.[8]

Something as simple as spending time in nature positively impacts our health, yet we are still destroying more and more of the natural world each day. We act like we have achieved utopia already, despite our inability to recognize, as a global society, something as simple as the value of our planet's natural resources.

We have forgotten the wisdom of our ancestors, and now we must try to relearn what we can, combining that with our knowledge and the technology at our fingertips. Only then will it be possible, as a society, to journey Beyond Domestication.

---

8   Bratman et al., 2015

PRACTICE 1

FOOD

THIS CHAPTER WILL look at four of the six kingdoms of food: Plants, Animals, Fungi and Bacteria. These four kingdoms make up the bulk of all food we eat, and having a relationship with each one is key to fostering health and well-being through diet.

The other two kingdoms that humans eat from are Protist and Archaea, but we will not be covering them in great detail. The Protist kingdom includes foods like seaweed, while the Archaea kingdom is made up of single-celled organisms, which can be similar to the bacteria foods we will look at.

We will start this chapter by looking at why I began my food journey and how the health of soil plays a role in food production. We will then explore each of the four kingdoms mentioned above before ending the chapter by looking at how human diets develop over time.

As I will point out regularly in this book, well-being is personal. What works for me may not work for you; similarly, what works for you may not work for me. The key throughout this book will be to play around with each of the Seven Practices, noticing what works for you.

Living With a Chronic Illness

Since I was diagnosed with Crohn's disease, I have had an interesting relationship with food. For those unfamiliar with either Crohn's or its partner in crime, Colitis, they are autoimmune diseases where your gut becomes inflamed, causing a wide range of side effects. Both of these diseases share symptoms with other bowel disorders such as IBS.

The NHS website states that Crohn's is a lifelong condition, which is what I was told. However, with NHS treatment and the rewilding of my lifestyle, I relieved my symptoms and achieved remission.

If you were a fly on the wall during my childhood, you may have expected that mealtimes could be overshadowed by the worry that I was either eating the wrong food or that I was going to trigger a flare-up of my Crohn's. But in reality, I felt pretty free to eat whatever I wanted without ever considering the idea that I could achieve remission. Like many children, I enjoyed junk food and fizzy drinks, even if they were a rarity and reserved for birthdays and Christmas.

Looking back now, I realize how lucky I was to have parents who limited my access to these sugary foods. And how lucky I was that even in the early 90s, my Mum had the presence of mind to question the quality of food available in supermarkets. I imagine that without her commitment to a healthier diet, I would not have been able to gain as much control over my disease as I have now—at least, it would have been much more difficult.

The food we ate was not perfect, but I still had access to various vegetables, fruits, and meats. As I grew up and left home, it became my responsibility to put food on my table, and like any good student, I took the cheapest path: frequenting dirty take-away joints and buying affordable frozen meals.

Unsurprisingly, my Crohn's symptoms were as prominent as ever throughout this time, although I was still oblivious to why that might be. It was not until I started a regular movement practice of running and going to the gym that I began to get back on track with my eating habits. I did not realize at the time that it would be the beginning of a long rewilding journey.

As soon as I challenged my eating habits and started to make changes, I saw improvements in my Crohn's symptoms. The more naturally I began to eat, the better I felt; it was as simple as that! This journey has taken us from sauerkraut to sourdough and everything in between.

In this food chapter, I want to share some of the stories and lessons that helped me on my rewilding journey.

Soil

If there is anything that does not get the appropriate credit it deserves for its role in our food, it is soil. Healthy soil is fundamental for food production and storing carbon underground, two vital steps in supporting a healthy human and planet. The future of humanity may be defined by our soil's future, with the current abuse of our farming land contributing to an overall degradation of global soil health.

Right now, a third of the planet's land has been degraded, with fertile soil being washed into the sea at a rate of over 24 billion tons yearly.[9] With food demands increasing, there appears to be

---

9   Soil Fertility and Erosion, 2014

no clear way to provide our environment with the break it needs to recover and rebuild.

Industrial agriculture, the backbone of our society, may currently be successful at feeding the ever-increasing populations, but it has been unable to foster the health of the planet alongside it.

Multiple yearly harvests and the aggressive use of agrochemicals have brought farming land around the globe to its knees. The knock-on effect being desertification and the relocation of the humans that once relied on that fertile soil.

We are now aware of the damage we are doing to the ground we rely on for so much of our food. There has never been a more critical time to act.

We are used to seeing large fields of monoculture plants growing; for years, this was the best practice. By monoculture, I mean the farmer's fields that are given over to just one crop at a time. However, we now know that our global ecosystems are not designed to host just one plant at once. One of the most significant damaging factors to our soil is the lack of diversity in the fields of our modern farms. This lack of diversity leads to soil erosion and an imbalance of nutrients in the soil.

To combat poor soil health, some farmers choose to work alongside nature to develop a natural solution to our human-engineered problem. One solution has been to plant a cover crop during winter when the fields are usually bare. These cover crops serve two purposes. On the one hand, they help improve the soil structure, leading to less erosion. And on the other hand, they also help capture and store vital nutrients like nitrogen from the air into the ground.[10] Another solution is to employ regenerative agriculture, which we will discuss later in this chapter.

How we interact with our soil will dictate the future of our planet. With the threat of desertification potentially making it impossible to farm in more parts of the globe, we have to ensure that we do our best now to protect the fertile land we still have.

As a consumer, all you can do is find as much information as possible about the origins of the food you buy.

Do you know what farm your meat came from?

Are the practices they are using to rear their animals destructive or productive?

What farm are your vegetables grown at?

Where possible, can you buy organic food or food with the Soil Association's quality mark? These are the questions we have to ask ourselves.

The future of farming will be unlikely to include single crops growing on vast fields due to the destruction this is causing. Chemical fertilizers and yearly ploughing cover the symptoms of a poor agricultural setup, but this can only last as long as our soil health. Time is running out.

Techniques like permaculture challenge farmers to let the natural world take its course alongside developing productive agricultural land. Can farmers use tools like permaculture to transform our entire understanding of food production?

We have to rewild our understanding of food production. As a society, we must be prepared to prioritize soil health and understand that the healthier our soil is, the healthier we will be.

---

10 What is soil health and why does it matter?, 2019

Food as Medicine

We have to think about how our food is grown, which makes sense. But it is not just about how our food is grown. It is about what we do to that food too.

In the last 200 years, the desire to synthesize plants into modern medicines has increased dramatically. In the 1820 edition of American Pharmacopoeia, 70 percent of drugs were still plant-based, compared to only 5.3 percent in 1950.[11] With the rise of synthetic medicines replacing plant-based medicines, we are ingesting synthetic drugs never before seen in the natural world for the first time.

On my well-being journey, I started considering the food I was eating to support my health and well-being the same way my Crohn's treatment was supposed to be. I stopped using my treatment as a reason to let me eat ultra-processed food and started to combine it with a healthy diet instead.

I did this because of the disconnection that has taken place over the last few hundred years between health and our food.

From traditional foods to supplements, the evolution of humanity has gone hand in hand with the evolution of diet, moving predominantly from wild foods foraged from the land to food manufactured through agriculture and now also factories.

When did we stop realizing that the food we eat can have as much impact on our health as medicine?

And what would happen if, every time we go to the doctors, their first question is, "Have you been eating well?"

---

11   Swain, 1972

The first time a doctor asked me about my diet was the first meeting after reaching remission when they finally asked me, "So, what *do* you actually eat then?"

I will never suggest that somebody stops taking prescribed medicine. I am merely trying to highlight the health benefits achievable through diet, not just medication.

My relationship with food has become a pursuit of what makes me feel well and healthy. I want to show that it is possible to foster a relationship with food that supports well-being.

Is it possible for us, as a society, to reconnect with our food in a way that supports health, well-being and our planet?

The one thing we do know for sure is that everybody is different. Each one of us is a combination of our unique genetics and life experiences. Even identical twins have different demands from their diets based purely on their different life experiences.[12]

For each of us, it can take a long time of trial and error before we finally feel comfortable with our diets. However, even with only a modicum of effort, it is possible to start experimenting and practicing with at least a wider variety of foods.

There is an opportunity for us to shun the more ultra-processed foods, which have become so popular over the last 50 years, favoring more healthy, sustainable whole foods. We have the chance right now to shake ourselves out of destructive agriculture, opting for regenerative agriculture.

Let's kick off our journey through the food kingdoms with our ancient friends, the plant.

---

12   Spector, 2017

PLANTS

Plants are experts of adaptation. For years, millions of humans across six of the seven continents have foraged from the unique diversity of plants in their area to provide food for themselves and their communities.

Across the globe today, there is a massive 390,900 different plant species on record, with 7,039 plants edible in some way.[13]

Domesticated Plants

With over 7,000 edible plants available worldwide, why are there only the same 15–25 vegetables on supermarket shelves year-round, year after year?

The average human in our society gets half of their calories from just three different crops: maize, rice and wheat. Compare that to the average neolithic hunter-gatherer, who consumed up to 300 plants yearly.

Why have we only heard about the same old fruit and vegetables our entire life? Since I was young, I have been eating more or less the same fruits: apples, bananas, grapes and oranges. And the same vegetables: broccoli, cauliflower, sprouts, peas and carrots.

Modern agriculture betrays how wide the variety of edible plants is, with more plant foraging taking place in the aisles of supermarkets these days than in the natural world. I also used to believe supermarkets contained all there was out there. In that way, I am glad to have suffered from Crohn's disease because if

---

13   Avis-Riordan, 2022

not, I may have never found the drive to start foraging wild plants to supplement my diet.

The small number of plants in our supermarkets are there because they were successfully domesticated for mass agriculture, favoring long life, uniform appearance and often a sweeter taste. Plant domestication has been occurring for 11,000 years alongside the domestication of humans and animals discussed in the introduction.

The first known domesticated plants were created by the community of people at Göbekli Tepe 11,000 years ago. These cereal-based plants represented the first step for our society down a long path of domestication. Since then, we have gone on to domesticate many other different plants.

Cabbage, brussels sprouts, kohlrabi, kale, broccoli and cauliflower are examples of veggies that were all domesticated from the same plant, *Brassica oleracea*.

Despite the downsides, the domestication of plants is one of the primary reasons why so many of us have widespread access to food. Our manipulation of plants has fed our population into the billions.

However, we have to take drastic action when preparing these crops for planting. Chemical fertilizers and weed killers are designed to destroy all organic life except for the crop species planted in the field. To ensure that the crops we want are capable of growing in that harsh environment, scientists are now opting to clone exact replicas of each plant to make sure that they can develop and grow amongst the destructive chemicals.

I believe this is a worrying development in our domestication journey with plants. The banana is one of the world's most successful crops, typically ranking in the top five for monetary value.

They are well known to be full of nutrients and are sold in nearly all food outlets worldwide. However, the success of the banana was not always so simple. The banana of the last 70 years that we know and love is, in fact, a clone.

Every banana most of us have ever eaten is an exact clone of another. That banana that you had in your lunchbox as a kid—cloned! That banana you had on your pancakes last weekend—cloned!

In the 1950s, United Fruit Company, the largest fruit manufacturer in America, started to refine the process of growing bananas. At this time, most bananas were grown across South and Central America.

To grow a standard product they began to clone one specific banana. Regardless of the difficulty and risk of moving to a monoculture, they finally cracked the code. United Fruit Company successfully developed a way of efficiently producing a banana that was never the wrong color, the wrong size or the wrong flavor.[14]

At the time, this was seen as a raging success, and for years that may have been the case. However, our reliance on this method of growing one banana also took us on a path that included the fruit's downfall for its use in commercial agriculture.

In only 15 years, the world's first cloned banana went commercially extinct. The Gros Michel, as it had been called upon invention in the 1950s, only survived until 1965 before being regarded as commercially extinct.

This commercial extinction occurred due to the international spreading of Panama disease, a fungal disease that could only be

---

14   Dunn, 2018

killed by burning any impacted crops.[15] In only 15 years, the top banana was wiped out by a global pandemic of Panama disease.

The banana industry quickly bounced back through the Cavendish strain of bananas. Despite being widely regarded as inferior to the Gros Michel, the Cavendish was blessed with immunity to the Panama disease, quickly becoming the new banana of choice.

However, as we saw in 1965, resting an entire industry's fate on a single cloned species can be a disastrous plan. When we rely on cloned plants, the whole food chain can be disrupted in no time if the wrong disease takes hold. And bad news for banana lovers, Panama disease is back!

Banana manufacturers have been trying to diversify since the 1980s, and there has been some success, but this success has not taken hold in the global market. The Cavendish banana still represents almost the totality of exports worldwide.

Like its predecessor, the Gros Michel, the Cavendish is threatened by a new strain of the Panama disease, TP4. This new strain was uncovered in Malaysia in 1990 and has since moved throughout South-East Asia and even jumped overseas to Australia and Africa.

With two of the significant landmasses heavily impacted by the spreading of TP4, it may only be a matter of time before we once again lose the top banana.

When you look at the ground zero for TP4 (Malaysia), it is interesting to note that this fungal disease was already present in Malaysian soil long before humans came along and started planting Cavendish bananas. TP4 is not a disease created at random to

---

15 Koeppel, 2009

smite agriculture's heroes. It is the product of natural evolution. If we had never dared to take a crop that originated in Africa and grow it in Asia, that fungal disease may never have been unable to work its way into the banana population.

Maximizing Nutrition

Domestication has allowed us to grow plants in greater and greater quantities, with these traits taming once wild plants into behaving like the crops we see today. However, for a plant to act that way is to go against its natural biology.

In the natural world, plants do not grow in the regimented lines of crops synonymous with our plant agriculture today. Wild plants are responsible for their survival, whereas domesticated plants rely on the human support systems of planting, weeding, fertilizing and general maintenance for their growth.

Our domesticated plants are now so tame that if a farmer left any agricultural fields, even for a week, he would risk losing his entire crop to pests or other competing plants (sometimes called weeds).

Our agricultural plants have lost many of their natural defenses against predators, and that trend looks to continue. With each year, it is becoming harder to coax domesticated plants from the land, adding to a large amount of labor already needed to make them grow. With soil health falling, we could be approaching a perfect storm for plant agriculture.

In an honest attempt to upscale our food production, we have created a system that relies on the degradation of the natural world for the opportunity to grow only a small handful of plants.

What makes this situation even worse is that the more a plant relies on humans for its survival, the fewer unique nutrients it is likely to pass into the food chain. When we domesticated the lettuce for our dinner tables, we created an almost entirely unrecognizable version compared to its wild progenitor.

The nutrients of a plant are primarily stored in its defense systems, and each time we get rid of the need for them to defend themselves, we lose vital nutritional aspects that are becoming harder and harder to replace in our diets.

One way to support health and well-being through diet is to ensure access to a wide range of nutrients from our food. The best way to do this without foraging is to put a wide range of fruits and vegetables on your plate. The goal here is to eat as broad and diverse a diet as possible, increasing the variety of vitamins that make it into your gut.

When I started my rewilding journey, one challenge to myself was to bring more bright fruits and vegetables high in phytonutrients into my diet. Blackberries, blueberries, and red cabbage all became staples in my fridge.

As with any well-being recommendation, you must find out what works for you, but you can do little wrong by eating a rainbow of bright-colored fruits and vegetables. Experiment with it and have fun. Try some new food!

One tip to help you identify how wild domesticated fruits are is to look for seeds. If a fruit you are eating does not have seeds that guarantees it comes from a long line of domesticated fruits, designed for ease of agriculture, not necessarily nutritional benefit.

Your Plant Journey

I would love to suggest that we all start foraging some of our food. But despite that being a good suggestion for health, the sheer volume of humans on this planet means that we would put wild foods at risk if we all started foraging regularly. Let alone the risks that may come from people accidentally eating the wrong food.

We can still benefit from fruit and vegetables found in shops (even if it can be a challenge to buy them ethically). Where I live in England, there will be no chance of me foraging an orange, for example. Although I do find plenty of nettles and blackberries. The future may still require mass-produced and cheap food sources. But these could be supplemented with local food, grown and harvested on a community level or foraged individually.

It is difficult to picture what the perfect relationship with plants looks like. Will we continue eating a lot of domesticated plants whilst making an effort to improve the diversity that reaches our table? Or will we start to look at wild plants again as having a widespread and valid contribution to our current diets?

There is no doubt that the future will have to include some form of mass-produced food, but when healthier, carbon-neutral food is freely available in our local area, we could be making a concerted effort to include it in our diets. Not only for our health but for the health of the planet too.

One way we can close the loop on plants is to grow our own. Nurture the soil in your area and grow food that makes it onto your plate and helps build resilience in your local food network.

This is the best way to ensure that our food comes from an ethical source and is good for us. When we grow our food, we control each stage in the plant's development, taking some pressure off of our agricultural system.

Another way is to consider the ingredients list of any processed food products you buy. Whether it is ketchup, muffins, bread, or biscuits, you can use the ingredients lists to ensure that you are not accidentally eating food that does not support healthy humans!

A simple tip is that if you do not understand what is on the ingredients list, then do not eat it. All the items I have listed above can be made from harmful, manufactured compounds that are used to extend shelf life and reduce manufacturing costs. Read the label and ditch anything that you do not understand. If in doubt, buy whole foods.

To learn about eating wild, book a foraging course in your area (with Beyond Domestication if you want to meet Amber and me). You will be amazed at the amount of tasty and medicinal food around you that you can incorporate into your diet.

What is stopping you? Eat bright, eat a variety, eat whole food and if possible, eat wild or grow your own! Take your tastebuds for a ride and maximize the nutrition in your diet.

ANIMALS

The animal food kingdom includes meat, fish, and other food items from an animal source, such as eggs, cheese, and milk.

Since humans domesticated the first sheep and goats in Southwest Asia between 11,000 and 10,000 years ago, our society has been readily harvesting animal proteins without needing to hunt.

This switch from hunting to agriculture is ongoing. Some hunter-gather societies (and some individuals within our society) still rely on hunted meats for a large portion of their diet. However, for most of us, it is now possible to get all of our animal products from agriculture.

Since domesticating the first sheep and goats, we have domesticated over 40 more land animals, 180 freshwater animals and 250 marine animals.[16] As we already know, plant domestication can drastically change a species' genetic profile, and it is no different for animals.

Meat Quality

Our reliance on farmed animals means that many humans are likely to go through their entire lives without eating a single wild animal product, unlike our ancestors, who only had access to meat from free, wild animals.

We have created a world where our society has access to endless farmed meats, to the point where we can now easily eat farmed meat for every meal.

But it was not always like this. In the early 1900s, meat from chickens was not a common part of the diet. Instead, chickens were raised for the eggs they produced as opposed to being raised for meat. A chicken would still be eaten once it reached the end of its egg-laying life, but the meat was not the priority.

This all began to change in 1944 when Howard C. Pierce, the poultry research director for the A&P Food Stores supermarket chain in the USA, proposed the development of a super-chicken with breasts the size of a turkey. The following summer, the

---

16   Bangun, Prajanto, Nusantoro, 2018

United States Department of Agriculture (USDA) launched the Chicken of Tomorrow contest.

Anyone could compete, with small farms, large farms and established companies granted a year to devise and breed a bird that would be more suitable to breed for meat.

In March 1948, 40 competing breeders shipped 720 eggs to a hatchery, where they were raised in purpose-built barns. The chicks were allowed to grow for 12 weeks before they were killed and judged. There were 18 criteria, including body structure, skin color and muscle development.

By June, the competition had a winner. Charles Vantress from California was awarded first place for his red-feathered hybrid of the New Hampshire chicken and a California strain of Cornish chicken.

Vantress won the competition again three years later with another crossbreed, further transforming the species into the chicken we most commonly eat today. The resilient, weather-tolerant chickens found in barnyards across America were now gone, replaced by the intricately bred hybrid birds.

The intricacies of raising these new chickens are similar to growing domesticated crops, where farmers rely on the provision of seeds from a supplier rather than developing their own. The Chicken of Tomorrow competition produced hybrid chickens that farmers could not successfully breed.

Raising hybrid chickens became like growing corn. Without the ability to breed their chicken, farmers had to return to the company each time to purchase new stock.[17]

---

17 Mckenna, 2018

The most commonly consumed chicken in the UK are the Ross and Cobb varieties; both descended from the Chicken of Tomorrow competition. The Ross can grow at such an unnatural pace that it would be the equivalent of a child weighing 392 pounds (28 stone) by its third birthday. It is typically reared indoors and slaughtered at 35 days old, by which time it can barely stand, let alone move.[18]

Our ability to disrupt the natural growth of the wild chicken into these manmade species provides food for humans, but at what cost to the chicken itself?

With so much meat available to us, it is down to us to prioritize the quality of meat we consume. Whether you buy directly from a farm or a shop, there are a few terms worth knowing that can help us make our choice.

Before we discuss the terms, it is worth considering the diets of the other animals we eat. Pigs and chickens are omnivores, which means they can eat plant and animal products. Compared to sheep, cows, and deer, that are classed as ruminant animals and eat only a diet of plants.

If we think about beef, the options available are either pasture-raised, grain-finished or grass-fed. Each of these describes a different diet eaten by the animal. Pasture-raised describes a diet of grass that is supplemented by grain. A decision that is typically made due to a lack of grass. Grain-finished describes a diet of grass up until harvest when they are fed grain and corn. Grass-fed describes a grass diet where animals are free to consume their natural diet for most of their lives.

---

18   O'Brien, 2017

Research on red meat in the diet discovered that the health benefits of both lamb and beef are greater when the animals consume a grass-only diet, their natural diet. In grass-fed beef and lamb, the ratio of omega 3 to omega 6 is higher, and the levels of saturated fat are a third of what we find in pasture-raised animals.[19]

There is a question of sustainability too. Grasslands are a crucial ecosystem across the globe, and ruminants like beef convert these inedible grasses into high-quality food for humans. Compare that to the pasture-raised or grain-finished animals that require grain to be grown by human hand at another farm, taking up additional space and travel costs.

Offal

Our current agricultural system has made us so familiar with specific cuts of meat that it is now possible to eat the same cut every day. Whether that is a beef steak, chicken thigh or pork mince, we no longer have the challenge of making use of an entire animal. We pick from the range we have, and that is that.

Even if we could diversify and have a different cut of meat, the chances are high that we would still be stuck with only the same 10–20 cuts of meat compared to the wider variety that our ancestors would have eaten.

A citizen of Victorian England with access to a lamb would never have discarded most of the animal to keep only the prime cuts: breast, thigh, and drumstick.

---

19   Wyness et al., 2011

Whilst those cuts would have been favored, the entire animal would have been used. The kidneys, liver, and heart are examples of lamb meat commonplace in our diets until only the last 70 years or so. The problem is that many health benefits can be found in the kidneys, liver and heart. Also known as offal.

We evolved into a world where we had the access and the necessity to utilize every possible part of an animal. Our bodies have evolved, over thousands of years, to expect the amino acids and nutrients this brings.[20]

Nose-to-tail eating is a simple way to unlock flavor, nutrients and potential cost-saving from your relationship with animal products. It supports the environment, too, as we maximize all of the meat from animals.

The Public Health Collaboration charity in the UK organizes Organuary, where they invite people to pledge to eat locally sourced organ meat twice a week or more.

Organuary promotes the benefits of bone marrow, heart, kidney, and liver, among other cuts of meat. Beef liver, in particular, is a great source of vitamins and minerals, such as B12, vitamin A, zinc, choline, folate, iron, and copper. Kidney contains many of the same benefits as liver, along with high amounts of selenium, supporting healthy kidney function. Who knew that eating kidney is good for your kidneys?[21]

Bone marrow is not organ meat but is still classed as offal and contains protein, B12, riboflavin and collagen. Collagen makes up 25–35 percent of the proteins in our body and is the

---

20 Nutritional Balance with Nose-to-Tail Eating—Jack Cincotta, 2020

21 Nutritional Benefits Of Organ Meats, 2022

main component of our connective tissues. Historically, humans received a great source of collagen from eating organ meats, ligaments, cartilage, and tendons. Whereas today, many people consume barely any.[22]

One of the easiest ways to consume bone marrow is as broth. People have been making bone broth for thousands of years, dating back to our prehistoric ancestors. Bone broth is made by boiling animal bones and connective tissue. This can either be used as stock for soups, sauces, gravy, or it can be drunk on its own.

When boiled, the collagen in the connective tissue is broken down into gelatin, glycine and glutamine, among other healthy amino acids.[23] Consuming just 300ml of bone broth has been shown to increase plasma levels of the amino acid glycine, which is required to form collagen in the human body.[24]

When was the last time you ate offal? If it was a long time ago, you might be missing out on some vital nutrients in your diet.

Modern Farming

The future of farming will look very different to our current approach, but the reality right now is that the farming of meat is still the primary way for our society to produce animal food products. However, that does not mean we must continue the same destructive agricultural practices we have utilized to get us to this point.

---

22 Axe, 2020
23 Paul, Leser and Oesser, 2019
24 Alcock, Shaw, Tee and Burke, 2019

Right now, farmers are experimenting with different methods of farming. Joel Salatin from Polyface Farms in Virginia, USA, has popularized unconventional farming methods with the goal of "emotionally, economically and environmentally enhancing agriculture." Joel has shown that by focusing on selling locally and building a relationship with his consumers, he can grow a thriving business without sacrificing his product's quality.

Joel's Polyface farm model has helped farmers across the USA provide affordable food without sacrificing biodiversity, whilst turning over a profit at the same time.

I will not pretend to be able to convey every nuance of how Joel manages Polyface farm, as the beauty truly lies in the detail of his work. But the premise is to provide land that allows animals to behave like they may have in the wild. The farm's ecosystem mimics nature's ecosystem.

Using modern technology like electric fencing, Joel rotates animals around his pasture, with each species of animal performing a unique task. For example, chickens are moved into a field on their portable shelter four days after the cows graze. This four-day delay gives flies on the cow manure time to pupate, providing free snacks for the chickens.

These free snacks, which only occur due to good farm management, end up providing 15 percent of the chicken's total diet. Not only does this provide cost-effective food for the chickens, it also organically distributes the manure left by the cows.

The net benefits of all Joel's innovations mean he can farm about four times as many cattle on his land as conventional farming allows. However, he did not stop there. The real cherry on the top comes from his drive to build a connection between farmer and consumer. Joel wants to drive food networks at a community level and has created his farm with that at the forefront. He does not sell to supermarkets or ship products over long distances; his meat is sold only to local businesses and people.

This last point is something that has grown in popularity all over the world, with modern consumers choosing to purchase food grown more locally.

Similar rewilding efforts are taking place in the UK. The Knepp Estate in Sussex used to be like most other farms. With government subsidies that propped up an unsustainable and inefficient farming system focused on growing large amounts of monoculture grains.

That was until their subsidies were cut in 2001, and their livelihoods were taken from them overnight. Since then, the innovative management team at Knepp has taken their estate on one of the most effective rewilding projects in the UK.

Similar to Joel Salatin's approach at Polyface farm, Knepp focused on mimicking the natural world as closely as possible and, where possible, opted to leave nature alone. An entire pasture was given back to the wild, and their livestock were gradually replaced with hardier species capable of being left well alone.

Instead of the traditional farming cow that we are used to seeing, they opted for longhorn cattle who could survive the cold winters unaided. Alongside the cattle, wild pigs and Exmoor ponies were given free rein to travel the estate, and between the three species, they began the long process of rewilding the damaged farmland.

Nowadays, Knepp has naturally become a haven for some of Europe's most endangered and elusive birds and insects. Scarce species like turtle doves, nightingales, peregrine falcons, and purple emperor butterflies now use Knepp as a breeding site.

Amber and I camped on Knepp in September of 2022, and there were points where over 50 storks would fly overhead. It was a scene like something from the African savannah. For Knepp to be capable of supporting so many large birds, along with all of its other biodiversity, is a positive sign for rewilding.

They have shown that by developing a functioning ecosystem, it is possible to repair the damage we have caused to our environment. Instead of keeping domesticated animals locked up in metal yards, we could encourage the cooperation of native cattle, horses and pigs and allow them to rewild our land as they have evolved to do.

Not only was Knepp able to rewild their land, but they were also able to convert their former cattle barns into office space, providing an alternative income as well as providing a natural haven for local businesses.

Imagine a world where our countryside is managed in the same way as Knepp. That would be a world where all currently unproductive and unused space is encouraged to rewild by the species that have evolved to live there. In early 2020, Knepp received permission to reintroduce the bison, a bovine species which was believed to have last roamed the UK 6,000 years ago. They will perform a similar role in the ecosystem to the longhorn cattle that they will now be living alongside, further solidifying the increased diversity and resilience in a now thriving part of the UK.

As consumers, we hold the power to drive this change. We vote every time we get our wallets out. By redistributing our spending towards healthier, regenerative sources of animal products, we are choosing to build a better world for us and the billions of other humans and animals we live alongside. You have a right to know exactly where your meat is coming from, and if the shop providing it does not know, it might be time to find a different place to shop.

While we must move forward, we can also look backwards if we want to improve the meat industry. It is time that we reconsider the butcher model, where you are only one link away from where your food is produced. And even better, what about cutting that link down and having a direct relationship with a farm? The internet has allowed farms like Joel Salatin's and many others to sell directly to consumers. Is there a farm or farmers market near you that offers products directly to the community?

We are all responsible for the change we wish to see. When we consciously try to learn where our meat is produced, we better understand our food. By buying and producing food more locally and, if possible, by altering our spending habits towards restorative and organic products, we may repair the fractured system currently in operation.

Currently, we are stuck between the necessity to feed a growing population and the need to introduce healthier animal products into society. People like Joel Salatin have proved that local production effectively brings resilience into our food chain. Now is the time for us, the consumer, to vote with our purchases and support the farmers in our area who are working for a better planet.

Can you choose to buy eggs from healthier, happier chickens? Or beef, from the cow, raised on the grass outside, rather than on grains? When we do this, we empower our farmers to give back areas of unproductive agricultural land to pasture to support both farmed and wild animals, which can all then feed into our food chain.

FUNGI

Long misunderstood, the humble fungi have a longer history than any of the plants or animals that make it to our dining table. Despite the USDA classifying the mushroom as a vegetable for nutritional purposes, they operate fundamentally, in a completely different manner to the chlorophyll-dependent plant family. Fungi, and the mushrooms they produce, are, without a doubt, in a whole kingdom of their own.

Fungi and plants have such a drastically different approach to life on Earth that the difference between the two is just as dramatic as the difference between plants and animals.

Instead of the cellulose in a plant cell, fungi function with chitin, a very different chemical. Plants grow by using cellulose to make glucose, a sugar used for energy; fungi grow by using chitin to build cell walls through a process of folding back on themselves to form chains.[25]

Mushrooms

When we are talking about fungi as food for the kitchen, we usually talk about mushrooms. A mushroom is a fungus that includes a *sporum*, also known as the fruiting body (even though fungi do not produce fruit).

These sporum are what we see growing in nature and packaged in our supermarkets. Out of five million recorded species of fungi, we have recorded over 10,000 as having mushroom sporum. These are just the species that have been recorded, and

---

25 Lenardon, Munro and Gow, 2010

it is believed there could be plenty more fungi with mushrooms unaccounted for.

The variety available in supermarkets is non-existent compared to the variety available to us in nature. Someone saying they do not eat mushrooms because of their experience with white button mushrooms is no different from saying they do not eat vegetables because they once tried broccoli and did not like it.

Fungi can also be used for more than just food. If you have ever had a serious illness or infection, fungi have likely already saved your life.

On September 28, 1928, Alexander Fleming witnessed a fungi colony killing any bacteria it came into contact with. This was the discovery of penicillin, the world's first antibiotic.[26]

We are learning more about the downside of antibiotics, but the downside of overuse still may not outweigh the negative impact if Fleming had never made that famous discovery. The fungus penicillin has saved millions of lives and is used worldwide to treat many illnesses, such as pneumonia and meningitis.

We know mushrooms have been part of the human diet for thousands of years. Archaeologists working in Spain at the El Mirón cave have found evidence of humans eating mushrooms as far back as 15,000 years ago. Dental testing of our Paleolithic predecessors in that region shows some form of fungi in their diets. The mushroom believed to have been consumed at the time is the bolete mushroom, widespread across Europe throughout much of history and pre-history. If you have eaten a porcini, you have eaten a bolete.[27]

---

26 Tan and Tatsumura, 2015

27 Power et al., 2015

It is reasonable to conclude that if mushrooms were being eaten 15,000 years ago by indigenous societies, they also appeared in our even more distant ancestors' diet. It only makes sense that as humans learned about the edible foods on their land, it would have been more a question of access than preference.

Only now, because of our access to other plant and animal foods, do we have the luxury of choosing not to eat from the fungi family. If you have been avoiding mushrooms in your diet, I invite you to explore this world more.

From a taste perspective, I recommend looking for oyster, porcini, chanterelle, chicken of the woods and parasol mushrooms. From a medicinal perspective, you may want to consider turkey tail, lions mane, reishi, cordyceps, chaga and shiitake mushrooms.

Never pick and eat a mushroom if you are not 100 percent sure you know what it is. If you are not 100 percent sure, leave it alone and definitely do not eat it. Amber and I attended multiple fungi foraging walks when we first started our journey with wild mushrooms, with our first find being turkey tails!

Stoned Ape Theory

To go even further down the mystery of fungi, I want to talk about a group of mushrooms that are long maligned but have seen a comeback since the late 2010s when they became the candidates for several unique scientific studies. Emerging from Terence Mckenna's Stoned Ape Theory, there is now a body of science that thinks our relationship with a specific species of mushrooms is so profound that it altered the future of the entire hominid family.

Of course, I am talking about psilocybin mushrooms, also known as psychotropic or psychedelic mushrooms. The American botanist Terrance McKenna hypothesized that these mushrooms might be the source of all consciousness. The idea is that these hallucinogens kick-started developments in creativity, language, and community, providing hominids with the consciousness that currently separates us from all other animals.

I do not talk about psychedelics lightly. Our society has built walls around the topic, whether on purpose or by accident, and I want to be careful about how I write this. However, no chapter on the role of fungi in society would be complete without recognizing the role of psilocybin in the development of consciousness.

It is difficult to pinpoint when humans started to consume psilocybin. Stone paintings from a Saharan aboriginal tribe in North Africa indicate psychedelic mushroom use as far back as 9,000 BC. But, as with the bolete mushroom, that was likely eaten earlier than the documented 15,000 years ago. Psilocybin use is also likely to have been present further back than the documented 9,000 years ago.

In three million years of hominid evolution, I would be surprised if we had only just got the handle on such a unique mushroom recently, especially when you consider Terrence Mckenna's hypothesis that our use of these unique psychedelics may have contributed to our development of consciousness.

Cleanup Crew

Our relationship with fungi touches so many different aspects of our life, from health and well-being to the root of consciousness itself. Despite all this, it still feels like science is playing catch up when it comes to the secrets of this wonderful fungi kingdom.

Each year it feels like there is another breakthrough in how we can use fungi in the future. One example from Kew Gardens is a report in 2018 that claims to have found a fungus that can break down plastics.[28]

Fungi have always been the cleanup crew of our world, devoting their existence to breaking down decaying compounds and returning them to the circle of life. And whilst you are reading this, scientists are working hard somewhere, alongside our fungi friends, to crack the code for breaking down the mountains of plastic found worldwide.

We all know plastics are one of the biggest threats to the biodiversity of life on Earth. Can science work alongside fungi in their efforts to break down plastic?

What if there are fungi available right now that would allow us to return harmful plastics to their pre-plastic state in a matter of weeks rather than hundreds of thousands of years?

Thankfully, we can anticipate that breakthroughs with this wonderful kingdom will continue. We learn more about fungi's intricate lives each year, and more mushrooms find themselves on our dinner plates. They are one of the keys to a healthy, diverse diet, and we can all make an effort to explore this exciting world some more.

If you are interested in wild mushrooms, you must take your first steps with a qualified professional. Only a small portion of

---

28   State of the World's Fungi, 2018

wild mushrooms are edible, and most require a basic understanding to identify safely. If you are ever questioning the mushroom you have picked, do not eat it!

BACTERIA

The final kingdom of food we will cover in detail in this book is bacteria. It may come as a surprise for some of you that I wanted to write about bacterial food like I am writing about eating plants, animals, and fungi. However, each year, we learn more about the importance of consuming healthy bacteria to aid health and well-being.

Microbiome

Much like the way animals inhabit the Earth, bacteria inhabit our gut. We can categorize these simplistically as good bacteria and harmful bacteria. Good bacteria work as stewards of our health, combatting illness by boosting immunity, and harmful bacteria work against us, causing illness and disease.

When we eat food that has been allowed to develop good bacteria, it can store itself in our gut, improving our biome's overall health.

Science is still opening doors into this world, and our understanding will continue to grow. But the information we already have tells us that it is becoming increasingly important to think about what makes the bacterial community inside us thrive.

The term used to describe the colony of bacteria in the human body is the microbiome. However, the human microbiome is home to more than bacteria, with other residents, including archaea, fungi, protists and viruses, forming part of the community. All of these coexist alongside our human cells.

It is difficult to comprehend the number of different bacteria inside us. Each human has their own unique range, which is dictated by genetics and their personal experiences in life. The food we eat affects the different bacteria in our microbiome, but it can also be affected by our lifestyle, genes, and medical history.

The first significant opportunity for our body to start building its colony of bacteria comes during birth. Babies born naturally are exposed to their mother's bacteria at birth. This is believed to stimulate the white blood cells to start ramping up the immune system and preparing the body for life outside the womb.

However, when babies are born by caesarean, they are not provided with this opportunity. This impact was not recognized until recently. When I was born by caesarean in 1991, I did not get the chance to benefit from this immune boost, as doctors still had limited knowledge of the biome.

Studies show that babies not born naturally are at a higher risk of developing obesity or diabetes due to the lack of exposure to their mother's bacteria at birth.[29] Fortunately, doctors are now aware of this and can expose newborn babies birthed by caesarean to their mother's bacteria straight after delivery.

It is scary to think how much we have learnt about how our biome operates during my lifetime alone, and it would be naive to believe that we do not have much more to learn. Situations like this make me wonder what else our society may innocently be doing that negatively impacts our biome, and consequently, our health.

---

29 Shao, Y. et al. 2019

Fermentation

For anybody that is now reflecting on their birth, do not fear! As important as it is for proper bacterial exposure during the early stage of our life, we can still expose ourselves to vital bacteria in later life by making the right food choices.

As we uncover more of our ancestors' secrets, it is clear that a massive part of food production was the preservation of foods whenever possible. Throughout history and prehistory, our ancestors accessed many bacterial foods through preservation, and one popular method of preservation that we still use today is fermentation.

Fermentation is the name given to a process that brings about a chemical change in bacteria. This process tends to make the fermented product more acidic, substantially increasing the food's shelf life.

In terms of our known history, archaeologists have even uncovered evidence of fermentation used to make beer as far back as 13,000 years ago in a prehistoric cave in Israel.[30] The exact origin of fermented food will likely forever remain unknown. But, considering fermentation's practicality as a tool to preserve food, I would be surprised if humans were not using this process even further back than 13,000 years ago. Especially considering that discoveries could have been made accidentally as food began to ferment naturally.

---

30 'World's oldest brewery' found in cave in Israel, say researchers, 2018

The consumption of fermented foods is now definitively linked to improvements in digestion and detoxification,[31] which explains why fermented foods such as kefir, sauerkraut and kombucha are popularized in the western diet. kefir, for example, can easily be added to the diet as the occasional yoghurt replacement.

Like most fermented foods, sauerkraut, typically made from cabbage, is high in probiotics, improving gut digestion. However, just like the milk on our shelves, if you buy it from the supermarket, it is likely to have been pasteurized for a longer shelf life.

When fermented food like sauerkraut is heated to the level of pasteurization, all the good and harmful bacteria end up dying. To make certain foods last longer on the shelves, we have to sacrifice some of the benefits that made them such good foods in the first place.

Just like supermarket sauerkraut, we are also pasteurizing our cow milk. As the distance between cow and consumer started to grow, pasteurization was used to stop the milk from curdling and prevent the growth of dangerous bacteria.

The term pasteurization came from Louis Pasteur, who, in the late 1800s, was the first scientist to determine the time and temperatures required to heat food to the point that microbes within it would be killed.[32]

At the time, the stress of widespread agricultural production led to diseases like tuberculosis being carried into the food chain by raw milk. Thankfully, the discovery that heating the milk could kill these harmful bacteria meant that humans could

---

31 Katz and Fallon Morell, 2016

32 HAAS, 1998

continue industrializing the dairy industry, keeping milk "fresher" for longer.

Pasteurization allowed humans to increase the safe distance that milk could travel before it turned, increasing the product's commercial viability. Unfortunately, what was not realized at the time was that along with killing the dangerous bacteria like tuberculosis or brucellosis (only present in the first place due to the increased distances between cow and consumer), the process of pasteurization was wiping out all of the good bacteria too.

This discovery did not stop some countries from implementing strict regulations on raw milk production. The regulations on selling raw milk are now so tight in certain countries that it is entirely illegal to sell raw milk to customers.

Fortunately, pasteurization has little impact on the nutritional value of the milk.[33] It is only the microbial content that suffers.

So, in that respect, we could continue our current relationship with pasteurized milk if we access bacterial foods from somewhere else. Unfortunately, we are also witnessing a microbial collapse in other parts of our food chain.

Sterile World

To understand a little more about our exposure to bacteria during our evolutionary history, researchers have spent time with hunter-gatherer tribes to see if their diets include a more comprehensive range of microbes than the typical domesticated diet.

---

33 MacDonald et al., 2011

Researcher and author Professor Tim Spector has gone to extreme lengths to document how exposure to different environments impacts the diversity of bacteria in our biome.

To learn more about our biome, Professor Spector spent three days living with the Hadza community, a hunter-gatherer tribe in Tanzania. During a project called MapMyGut, the Hadza were discovered as having one of the most diverse ranges of different species inhabiting their biome, and the idea was to find out the extent to which another humans biome (in this case, Professor Spector) may change during a short stay with the Hadza.

The three days Professor Spector spent with the Hadza were organized to be as intensive as possible, with the Professor exposed to as many natural behaviors of the Hadza people as possible. By regularly recording his stool samples to analyze back in London, Professor Spector scientifically showed clear differences in his microbiome's quality from the time he spent with the tribe compared to his normal biome.

Professor Spector's time with the Hadza caused his overall microbe diversity to go up by a massive 20 percent! Showing that our gut custodians can be heavily impacted by the food we choose to eat. However, it was not to last, and after only a few days in his regular lifestyle, the diversity had gone back down to the level it was before the trip.

Whether Professor Spector could keep a small amount of diversity is hard to tell, as microbe levels fluctuate up and down naturally. However, it showed that time spent eating a wilder diet diversified his microbiome, potentially supporting positive health and well-being.[34]

---

34 Spector, 2017

The Hadza have been seen to eat over 600 different species of plants and animals each year, a major difference from the 100–150 species available to our society through agriculture.

We are moving towards a sterile world for all the right reasons, but we fail to recognize the unexpected consequences. Consequences that, if left unchecked, could lead to significant drawbacks in the microbial levels found in our food.

Scientists at the Institute of Cancer Research London now believe that infants living in overly sterile homes could even be more at risk of developing illnesses. One of the leading leukaemia biologists, Professor Sir Mel Greaves, says, "The problem is not infection, the problem is lack of infection."[35]

We are only just realizing the gravity of building such a sterile world around us. Right now, it is time for us to recognize that the world our predecessors have created is coddling the human body, protecting it from not only harmful bacteria but all of the helpful necessary bacteria too.

All of these changes have been for the right reasons, limiting the spread of serious diseases. But we must recognize the role that fermented foods play in a healthy human diet.

As we have gained the technology to micromanage the land of entire countries, as seen throughout England (and many other countries), we have created sterile agricultural and distribution processes. With the surface of England now used mostly for monoculture crops, there have been significant losses among insect, fungi and bacterial species that rely on decay. Most of our current national and global agricultural systems are destroying

35   Bosely, 2018

the natural life support systems that have fostered life up to this point.

DIET

All is not lost. We are a remarkably adaptable species, and as we have evolved, we have developed the capacity to convert energy from new food items as they become available.

You Are What Your Ancestors Ate

I spoke about the differences between milk and raw milk earlier. However, milk consumption, on the whole, is still one of the most recent foods that humans have started to consume. The consumption of milk in the human diet can be traced back to 7,500 years ago.[36] It is assumed that as farmers in western Europe started domesticating livestock, they also began to consume any additional by-products provided by that livestock. In this case, dairy.

Lactose intolerance is when people cannot effectively process food produced from dairy. By looking at the rates of lactose intolerance around the world, you can tell which parts of the world have been consuming animal milk the longest, as they have the biggest portion of lactose-tolerant citizens. For example, a typical individual in Sweden is likely to have only a 4 percent chance of lactose intolerance. In contrast, an individual's typical nutritional

---

36   Marshall, 2019

profile in China is likely to have a 90 percent chance of being intolerant to lactose.[37]

What this shows is that the human body is capable of massive diet adaption over time. The theory of evolution would suggest that as farmers in western Europe started feeding their families lactose-based diets, any lactose-intolerant individuals in that population would have been less likely to survive and pass on their genes. Over time, this slowly created a lactose tolerant populous. I am not suggesting that we start selectively breeding for lactose tolerance, but I am using this example to highlight how we have adapted over time.

Recently there have been efforts among the health-conscious to mimic the diets of our wild ancestors. Popular examples include the paleo diet, which restricts all your food options to those that humans had access to in the Paleolithic era (the era that covers the period when hominids were first active on the Earth's surface, circa three million years ago, up to the start of the agricultural revolution, 11,000 years ago).

Eating a paleo diet means restricting all domesticated cereal grains, legumes, dairy, potatoes, and other refined or processed foods. In my experience, my time spent experimenting with the paleo diet did not significantly impact my health as I was already on a diet focused on eating whole foods. I also know from experimentation that my body does well eating dairy, so over time, I included it as a part of my diet despite the paleo restrictions.

We are learning so much about diet each year that we must become lifetime learners of food. Thanks in no small part to Sally

---

37   Map of Milk Consumption & Lactose Intolerance Around the World, 2012

Norton's book Toxic Superfoods, I have recently changed my own opinion about certain foods I regularly ate after learning about the role of oxalates in our diet.

Oxalates are organic compounds found in high numbers in plants such as spinach, rhubarb, cinnamon and chia seeds. In the wild, high-oxalate plants would have either been entirely inedible or available seasonally, limiting the ability for the compounds to build up in the body. However, modern agriculture makes oxalates available to us in high doses all year round.

High-oxalate diets have become so common that restriction of high-oxalate food can be used as therapy for recurrent kidney stones[38] and calcium oxalate-caused arthritis.[39]

It is not always possible to just listen to experts and find the answers to your well-being. You must reflect on your diet and, if necessary, make changes. We are a product of our unique genetics and experiences, and our diets reflect that. What works for you will be personal.

Fasting

It is a challenge to highlight any one thing that helped me achieve remission from Crohn's disease. However, if I had to pick one related to food, it might be fasting.

To this day, I still practice intermittent fasting, eating only within an eight-hour window. Usually that is between 12 pm–8 pm. I allow myself the occasional day off, but most days, I give my gut the chance to have 16 hours of rest.

---

38   Massey et al., 1993

39   Lorenz et al., 2013

Our bodies have evolved to go without food, and our all-day, everyday access to food is debilitating for our gut. It is undoubtedly a good thing to have access to food, but we must not let it take over our health.

If you are like me before I started fasting, you have probably never let your gut have the rest it needs. Think about the last time you did not eat for 16 hours. Do you even remember when that was?

You can ease yourself into fasting. You do not need to start with a 16-hour fast on day one. Any attempt to go beyond your normal fasted time will condition your body to become comfortable in a fasted state. Try moving your breakfast back a couple of hours or your dinner forward a couple of hours. The goal always being to increase the amount of time between eating.

I invite everybody reading this to give it a go. You can still drink water and tea (without milk). Every time we choose to fast, we give our body the chance to burn through our sugar reserves and get into our fat reserves, leading to a longer life, leaner figure and a sharper mind.[40]

Personally, Amber and I want to take more of an active responsibility in our relationship with food. We want to find a sense of place created by the food around us. We do not want to rely on hyper-processed, chemically sprayed food when there may be a more nutrient-dense local option growing nearby.

The fact that all wild foods are grown using free solar and water only adds to their value and is another reason to consider

---

40 de Cabo and Mattson, 2019

their role in your diet. I practice foraging and archery with the aim that one day I will be able to support my health with wild foods. For me, it is about having control of my future. I know it is not easy whilst I live in London, and my next journey will be to find a space in this world where self-sustainability is still possible.

When eating wild, you are choosing to embrace not just the quality of your life but the quality of the life you are eating from. To be alive is to take life, and eating wild allows you to eat animals, plants and fungi grown and harvested as nature intended.

Where possible, I would much rather ethically harvest wild animals, plants and mushooms than contribute to the destructive and unethical agriculture of animals and plants that experience a life of suffering and frustration.

This is a personal choice for my life and an insight into how I want to build my relationship with food, but it is not the only way.

Remember that when you begin your journey with wild food, it may take time before your taste buds adapt.

I remember how bitter garlic mustard tasted the first time I foraged it. My tastebuds were still adapted to a high-sugar diet. However, my body now yearns for the bitterness in these wild plants as I have reduced the amount of sugar in my diet.

Until you decide to reduce the junk food in your diet, your body may always cling to the desire for those sugary treats.

The future of healthy eating will include a combination of all four kingdoms we have looked at. At a personal level, health and well-being can be considered by simply looking at diet and trying to minimize ultra-processed foods whilst eating a variety of fruits, vegetables and mushrooms alongside animal products. Remember, whole ingredients over processed options!

We can play our own part in that journey by challenging our food stores to inform us where the food is from. When you are shopping, can you ask the following questions:

Where did the food come from?

Who grew it?

Is the food grown ethically?

If the food shop cannot answer these simple questions, should we buy their food?

Seven Practice Recommendations

- Forage and eat wild food
- Grow your own food
- Include offal in your diet
- Eat a species of mushroom you have not had before
- Try fermented food
- Cook a meal using only wholefoods
- Let the body fast for over 16 hours

PRACTICE 2

WATER

YOU CAN TURN on a tap in most countries worldwide, from Argentina to France, and you will be typically greeted with clean, drinkable water. When you look at our major cities, they have all developed around natural water. Water that was used for drinking, cleaning, cooking and transportation.

Of course, many countries still lack this basic need, with millions of people relying on other methods for their drinking water. Before tap water, everyone relied on the wild and natural water systems that flow over Earth.

Prerequisite for Life

The oceans cover roughly 70 percent of the Earth's surface, with humans still having explored less of the ocean floor than the moon. Water is not just a prerequisite for human life. It is a prerequisite for all life on Earth.

The first organisms to break the water's surface all those millions of years ago and populate the land became the early ancestors of the modern plants and insects we know today. It was one-way traffic from there, as plants, animals, fungi, and bacteria spread their roots, legs, and wings across the vast empty continents of Earth.

However, we have not forgotten our water-based origins. The human body is around 60 percent water (varying between genders and ages) and uses water as the primary building block of our cells. Water also plays a critical role in many other bodily functions, such as eating and processing food.

DRINKING WATER

As with the domestication of plants and animals, we have also tried to domesticate our water. In many countries, we have interrupted natural water flows on a large scale by building dams and reservoirs that provide water and electricity for us.

Modern countries across the globe are all now capable of providing access to clean water through the public water supply. Houses in rural areas may still access their water straight from a spring or a deep well. But the primary way to access water in the 21st century is to pay a water company to provide you with water that they have treated.

Aqueducts

We must go back to the days of the Romans to see the first known significant impact that our society had on the natural processes of water.

One of the many significant engineering breakthroughs of the Romans was their aqueduct technology. An aqueduct can carry water for many miles, making it possible for clean water to be accessible in previously impossible locations.

As populations grew, it was no longer necessary for them to split when the strain on natural water became too high. They could now build aqueducts, and water would simply be piped in from elsewhere.

The first aqueduct in Rome was finished in 312BC and measured 16,445 meters in length. The Appia aqueduct, as it became known, was an early sign that our society had the means to change our environment radically.[41]

Their invention was a solution to the health problems caused by unclean water, as the traditional water sources of natural springs, wells and rivers became dirtied by overpopulation. These days most water companies rely solely on a mix of surface water and groundwater to supply our homes. Groundwater is accessed by drilling down into the Earth to reach water stored in veins under the ground, similar to how a well works. Surface water is water that falls as rain and is collected before it reaches the sea via streams and rivers.

Nowadays, the surface water (rivers, streams etc.) in many developed countries is becoming undrinkable. Places where our ancestors may have safely drunk throughout their lives are now heavily treated because of concerns about water quality.

Surface water supplies 60 percent of the water in the US.[42] Our governments have to ensure that contamination from sewage, urban and rural surface runoff and pharmaceutical chemicals are managed safely, so we do not contaminate the water that comes from our taps.

---

41 Gill, 2018

42 Dieter and Maupin, 2015

I am not suggesting that water flowing 20,000 years ago was completely free of harmful organisms. In our wild past, surface water running in rivers and streams would have likely included harmful organisms, potentially due to something like a dead animal in the water upstream. However, the health risk is likely significantly lower than today. As we saw during the section on bacterial food, exposure to bacteria may have also benefited the biome of our ancient ancestors.

Groundwater is protected from the tampering of our society. Groundwater is not only the most natural form of water left available to all life on Earth but may also be the most natural substance left. The industrial revolution has cut deep scars across the face of our planet. Scars so deep that the presence of unnatural chemicals is now found in areas as wild as Antarctica.

However, in many places, groundwater has been protected under the Earth's surface for so long that it may now be the last way to truly expose ourselves to a substance that has not been a victim of any industrialization by humans.

All of us can cut out the proverbial middleman by collecting our own groundwater. My goal is to live in a place where we can collect natural water directly from a local spring. When in that place, we will collect and store the spring water in glass bottles to use just as we do tap water now.

St Ann's Well is a spring in the center of Buxton in the Peak District, UK, where warm water has flowed continuously for centuries. It is a well-known spot that locals use to access clean groundwater all year round. Can you find a similar spot near where you live?

For those interested in finding your local spring, there is a great website, www.findaspring.com, that lists many waterholes all around the globe. This website was founded by one of my rewilding heroes, Daniel Vitalis. Daniel started the website as a way of helping people to access groundwater.

Plastic Bottles

If you do not have access to a local spring, in most places tap water is still preferable to plastic bottled water! I choose to drink tap water over plastic bottled water on almost every occasion.

In the parts of the world where we are struggling to provide clean surface or groundwater for people to drink, bottled water may be the only solution. But there are risks associated with drinking from plastic bottles.

Despite the increased cost, two destructive things that are clear about bottled water are the extravagant carbon footprint required to produce a bottle and the risk of microplastics remaining in the human body and on the planet after use.

Water stored in plastic bottles, especially those containing BPA, has the potential to be harmful to us when consumed. Dr Kellogg Schwab, director of the Johns Hopkins University Water Institute, says, "A chemical called bisphenol-A, or BPA, along with other things used to manufacture plastic, can leach into your water if the bottle heats up or sits in the sun."

The side effects of this leaching are severe, with consumption of BPA leading to an increased risk of heart disease or cancer. Just think, every time you have grabbed plastic bottled water off the shelf in a shop, you may have consumed harmful plastics without knowing it.[43]

---

43 Heid, 2014

An easy way to avoid unnecessary plastic entering our bodies is to carry a reusable bottle. Obviously not a plastic one. Many of us can all do more to reduce our single-use plastic impact, and refilling instead of buying new will go a long way to saving the planet and your wallet.

We use simple stainless-steel bottles that can be easily cleaned. Make sure you get a double-walled bottle for hot drinks, so you can still pick it up after!

Carrying a non-plastic reusable bottle is not the only thing we can do to improve our relationship with drinking water.

Make a date with water one of the first things you do every morning. Each night as we respirate in sleep, we exhale water vapor. After a full night's sleep, we are left with a water debt to pay if we want our brain and body to work at their best.

If you want to stop treating yourself to sugary drinks, it is easier to kick the habit if you keep hydrated. When you feel the urge to drink a fruit juice, cola, or other sugary drink, it can be your body telling you it is dehydrated. That is why orange juice tastes so nice in the morning.

The next time you feel the urge for sugary drinks, drink half a liter of water and wait 10 minutes to see if you still want that sugary treat. Hopefully, your urge will have gone!

SWIMMING

Our waterways have been used by humans for centuries before we built the first aqueduct. Whether for travel, food, or cleaning, we have lived alongside wild water for much of our evolution.

Humans are well adapted for life alongside water, and we are seeing many people reconnecting to nature through the lens of wild swimming.

Wild Swimming

This return to wild swimming is picking up speed in the UK, with Sports England revealing that over 4.1 million Brits swam in lakes, rivers and seas between November 2017 and November 2018. The media has also taken to wild swimming, with popular work written on the sanctity of the ladies' pond at Hampstead Heath in London.

Membership to the Outdoor Swimming Society in England grew by a third in 2020, with Swim England counting the 2.1 million people who preferred to swim in wild water in 2019.[44]

The culture of wild swimming in the UK has been for landowners to simply say no, and it is taking time to change that stance. With England and Wales, two of the few nations globally to privatize their Water Companies, even many of their reservoirs have been made off limits for swimmers, with preferences given to sailing and fishing.

We can continue to educate ourselves about the risks and make informed decisions about the safety of our wild swimming spots rather than just relying on the blanket rule that swimming cannot take place safely. We can work with landowners to show that when people engage with a landscape, in this case, a swimming spot, they are more driven to look after it too.

---

44 Coldwell, 2021

When wild swimming in an unsupervised spot without lifeguards, ensure you have an idea of any moving water and currents. Swimming with friends is a great way to have support around you if it is needed. I am also mindful to pick out a nice safe spot where I can slip in and out of the water easily.

Reconnecting to nature is a great reason to swim in wild water, and there are other benefits to taking a dip in our wild waterways too.

Cold Shock Protein

When we swim in natural water, we do not get the luxury of heating it to our desired temperatures. We are at the whim of the season, just like our ancestors would have been. This can mean exposing our bodies to some chilling cold water.

When we slip into cold water, our body generates cold shock proteins. This is triggered by our body reacting to the stress of the cold. Now, this may sound like an acute kind of hell to many readers. An ice bath is not everybody's idea of a relaxing afternoon. But cold shock proteins in the body are now considered an indication of protection from various diseases such as cancer, Alzheimer's, and dementia.[45]

There is a long road of research ahead as we unpack exactly how cold shock protein expression impacts the human body. However, cold dips are not a fad. They are becoming a real weapon in the arsenal of self-care.

I know the challenge of beginning a journey with cold water and can say to anybody starting out that it does get better! We

---

45 Lindquist and Mertens, 2018

will learn from Kevin O'Neill, also known as Breatheolution, in the next chapter how to use our breath to keep us in the cold for longer.

Overcoming my fear of the cold came more recently in my rewilding journey and has enabled me to swim throughout the year in many beautiful spots. I can embrace the physical health and raw feeling of having overcome a challenge.

This movement has coincided with the success of people like Wim Hof—the record-breaking Iceman. Wim is a practitioner of ice treatment, exposing his body to ice water to boost his body's immune system. We will discuss Wim's groundbreaking work in the chapter on Air. But the practice of cold water immersion is quickly gaining popularity for both health and community reasons.

If a cold bath or dip are not at the top of your rewilding priorities, then treat yourself to the opposite, a warm bath. We can benefit from hot shock proteins with a hot bath able to stimulate the body in a similar way to a cold one. A mindful warm bath after a long day is a great way to relax and prepare for a healthy night's sleep.

We are surrounded by so many ways to immerse ourselves in water. And as beings that evolved from water (and are still made up predominantly of water), we may always be drawn to areas of open water. A planet without water is a planet without life as we know it.

Our society makes it easy to consider water an infinite resource, but that is not the case. Treat every time you turn on the tap as a gift. Find those heavenly natural water spots and go in for a dip whilst you still can.

WATER ON THE LAND

Globally, the water table is suffering; it is falling from Canada to India and Iceland to Australia. Of the world's 37 major aquifers (a body of rock that contains groundwater), 21 are now receding.[46]

The abuse of water by our society is on the brink of causing a major catastrophe. The idea that entire cities may one day wake up to find no water coming from their taps is a real possibility in our lifetime.

Deforestation

In 2019, scientists led an expedition into the Amazon jungle to try and understand why the water table located there was falling so much. They found that the construction of hydropower dams alongside deforestation was causing the water table to recede.

However, it was not until scientists were able to analyze images over time that they realized the true scale of the problem. Satellite images taken over 33 years (from 1985 to 2017) showed the changing state of the Amazon's surface water, with a staggering 350km2 of surface freshwater lost each year.[47]

The damage is most prominent in an area of the southern Amazon known as the "deforestation arch." The most impacted areas are the floodplains and lagoons, typically breeding grounds for a myriad of species such as freshwater dolphins, fish, and turtles. Because of the impact of humans, entire breeding sites are believed to be lost, with the knock-on effects on the animals

---

46 Smedley, 2017

47 Souza et al., 2019

(and humans) reliant on those populations yet to be clearly understood.

The vast wealth of knowledge held by the animals, plants, fungi, and bacteria that, in many cases, exist only in the Amazon is something that we are currently unable to comprehend. In the grand scheme of human activity, we only recently invented the technology to begin a scientific analysis of the incredible biodiversity held by this ancient rainforest. We have also lost generations of the Amazon's indigenous knowledge during the great forgetting. It is up to us to ensure that future generations can keep learning from this incredible environment by finding ways to work together with the natural order rather than against it.

We are seeing something similar across different parts of the world with the same destruction of the water table happening in Madagascar.

Satellite imagery again makes it possible to see the scale of the damage. The land visibly changes color as the surface water runs off into rivers, taking any loose soil with it. Deforestation (among other things) is putting surface water at risk and damaging the soil that we rely on for our food. There may be a point soon where deforestation in some parts of the world has been so severe for so long that even if we wanted the environment to recover, there would no longer be enough nutrient-dense soil.[48]

It is not just the jungles where we have upset the natural balance. We see similar signs across all of the modern world. Global flooding and extreme rainfall have increased by over 50 percent in the last decade alone.[49]

---

48 Erosion in Madagascar, n.d.

49 Hov, Cubasch and Fischer, 2013

Ironically, major cities worldwide are now at risk of flooding from the very surface water that facilitated the city's development in the first place. It is the perfect storm. The warming of the world's climate is melting more ice than typical, and the land we have left is storing less water than it is capable of. All of this is culminating in rising sea levels.

Looking at the numbers of people living in coastal cities makes the process of risk managing rising water levels seem even more vital. The coastal cities of Guangzhou with 14 million inhabitants, Mumbai with 12 million inhabitants and Osaka with 20 million inhabitants all stand to lose substantial amounts of habitable land if the sea level rises as predicted.[50]

A study published by Nature estimates that the homes of 300 million people will suffer a severe flood at least once before 2050. This indicates a significant jump from the previous estimation of 80 million people.[51]

Things do not look much better back in Europe. In the UK, compound flooding (where heavy rain combines with severe storms) is predicted to cause major damage to seaside areas such as Devon and Cornwall in the next few years.

Things get even worse for the citizens of mainland Europe. Currently, the areas most impacted by compound flooding are located in the Mediterranean, with the gulf of Valencia, Algeria, the gulf of Lyon and southern Turkey, all thought to be at risk of severe weather events. However, as global warming increases,

---

50 Cassidy, 2018
51 Kulp and Strauss, 2019

these events will move further up the coast, impacting populations on the North Sea's east and west coasts.[52]

It is not just our climate abuse that has put us in the firing line
for increased flooding. The way we treat the land we still have is
also playing right into the hands of climate disasters.

We have already seen that deforestation in two major jungles
is leading to a loss of nutrient-dense soil as there are no trees
to stop the soil from running off with the surface water into
the oceans.

This is exactly the same predicament that people are facing
in the UK. The only difference between these two situations is
that the loss of trees from our world's rainforests is recent while
the trees of Great Britain are long gone. It has been 2000 years
since the Romans first rolled through and domesticated the native
druids of Britain with the introduction of agriculture. In that
short time, the small island's population has multiplied countless
times, leading to wild and natural land being diverted for use by
our society.

As with any growing population in our society, the land tends
to be sacrificed to support the agriculture that feeds new mouths.
Throughout our story, countless acres of ancient forests have been
displaced for the sake of grains and sheep. These ancient forests
that were capable of predicting weather patterns and holding
on to more water in times of increased surface water may have
held the key to coping with fluctuating and potentially damaging
rainfall.

However, it is not just as simple as replanting the forests. The
ability of the trees to adapt to fluctuating weather patterns is a

---

52 McGrath, 2019

learned ability, passed down from tree to sapling over 100s of generations. Every time we cut down an ancient woodland anywhere in the world, we are losing the intelligence of a place, along with the countless fungi and invertebrate species that may be unique to that specific area.

The UK is an excellent example of a country that has undergone a profound change as different keystone species have been lost.

In a country that has completely wiped out natural predators, we have seen the takeover of previously predated species like deer. The highlands of Scotland are a perfect example of land suffering from overgrazing. In Britain, the red deer are the possession of nobody. However, if they are grazing and living on your land, you are expected to assume responsibility for their management. There are estimated to now be over 1.5 million deer residing throughout the UK. In the Cairngorms National Park in the heart of Scotland, packs of deer 1,000 strong have been known to roam.

In Glen Affric, the charity Trees have been planting native tree corridors between Scotland's west and east coasts, connecting the remaining sections of the ancient Caledonian Forest. However, when the deer fences were damaged by heavy snowfall, the red deer broke into the tree corridor and munched their way happily through a decade of work.[53]

I am not saying the deer is to blame. They are simply acting on instinct. Without any natural wild predator on the land, they have very little to be scared of and can roam unchecked. But, when allowed to roam in the numbers they do, there is no chance for the trees to return.

---

53   Flyn, 2018

Beavers

You would be excused for being surprised by the presence of the beaver in a chapter about rewilding our well-being with water. However, the story of the beaver is linked closely to the health of many waterways across Europe and North America.

Just like the auroch we discussed in the introduction, beavers are a keystone species in the ecosystems where they operate. When beavers thrive, the whole ecosystem has a bigger chance to thrive. We can see the impact that beavers have had by looking at where they have been reintroduced in the UK.

In early 2020, the UK was hit by Storm Ciara and Storm Dennis in the space of a week and some areas were wholly devastated by the dramatic weather that came in such a short period. It is a bad sign when a storm even has to be named, implying that we are experiencing a significant storm. To have faced two in such a short time highlights the increased turbulence that our weather patterns are experiencing.

The aftermath of Storm Caira and Dennis left scientists in the UK considering the standards of water management systems. With increased flooding showing no signs of abating, there is an increased urgency to invest more in water defenses.

The UK has been insistent on taking the fight to nature, building bigger walls, and constructing industrial dams upriver of towns most at risk of flooding. However, there is now the need to take a different approach.

The good news is that both of these storms showed the impact that new colonies of beavers, a previously missing keystone species, have in minimizing water damage.

There are a couple of well-documented areas in the UK that have been allowed to rewild, encouraging natural water movement over the land.

The beginning of 2020 was met with the green light from the UK government for further reintroduction of beavers at key points in the country. The reintroduction of beavers was allowed to continue due to the success of beavers in locations such as Bamff in Scotland and Cropton Forest in England. The dams they built not just fostered the development of young mammals and fish but have also played a significant role in holding back large surges of water moving down river.

The beavers of Bamff were originally escapees from a captive population, and they slowly grew in influence over the landscape as they reproduced. However, the beavers at Cropton Forest were introduced by conservationists to see if their water management practices could complement current flood prevention measures. Starting in 2019, this was the first official study in the UK and was the first time since the last wild beaver was killed in the 16th century that the UK government has attempted to address this imbalance.[54]

So how did the beavers in Cropton Forest do when Storm Caira and Dennis came along? Early considerations are that the impact of the beaver's water management was vital in preventing flooding, with the beavers getting straight to work and building a large dam that connected the river with its floodplain.

Cath Bashforth, an ecologist from Forestry England for Yorkshire, said: "The beavers have been busy and made a large dam in the river. They have also fixed 'leaks' in ponds, meaning more

---

54 Barnett, 2019

water is being stored in them. Their activity has made a difference in how the water moves through the enclosure. The dam appears to be reconnecting the river to its floodplain."[55]

Our relationship with water is an intimate one. We have evolved alongside this gift from Earth. Modern humans do not have to go a day or even a morning without water.

The beaver has shown us that it is possible to work smarter, not harder. Yes, they may cause flooding damage to areas built on historic floodplains, but this is all part of finding our society's balance with the natural world. It is up to us to carve the path forward for our planet and the water systems that flow across it. We can only enjoy wild swimming and spring water if we continue to have access to it. Our waterways were here before us and will be here long after humans are gone, and it is up to us to ensure that we work alongside this force of nature rather than against it.

Seven Practice Recommendations

- Drink water first thing
- Find a spring and drink from it
- Avoid water packaged in plastic
- Carry a reusable bottle
- Swim in natural water
- Try a cold water dip
- Have a warm bath before bed

---

55 Newton, 2020

AIR

THE AIR WE breathe is made up of a mixture of various elements, which over time have been recorded to fluctuate and change, drastically altering the life that thrives on our planet. Scientists have been able to look at fossil records and determine when these changes occurred to further understand our home's prehistory.

Currently, the air in our atmosphere is made up of nitrogen, oxygen, and argon. The amounts vary, but we expect about 78 percent nitrogen and 21 percent oxygen, with the remaining 1 percent made up of carbon dioxide, argon, and other minor gasses.

Just as all life on Earth requires water, we also require air. However, it is not just the presence of oxygen that has allowed humans to evolve over the last three million years; we also require a specific percentage of oxygen in the air.

Climate Change

Over 300 million years ago, the world was a completely different place. Imagine walking through North America at the time.

There would be no bison, birds or wolves. Instead, you would witness amphibious vertebrates up to 20 feet in length and larger-than-life arthropods (picture massive water-reptile bears and dragonflies as big as a bird of prey). These animals lived in the land of swamps, swamps that were filled with club moss the size of trees.

This alien stage in the evolution of life on Earth was due to a new development in the evolution of plants. Plants evolved to produce a new chemical compound called lignin, a compound used to build plants up, more commonly known as wood.

However, the bacteria and fungi present on Earth at the time were not ready for this stage in plant evolution and, for years, could not decompose any wood on the planet. As bacteria uses oxygen in the air to break down the carbon-based plants, the inability to break down the newly evolved wood led to increased oxygen in the air. It also led to undecomposed wood becoming coal over thousands of years.

Eventually, the bacteria and fungi of Earth cracked the code and were able to start breaking down wood back into its organic compounds.

A mass extinction ended this period of evolution on Earth. There is not a clear understanding of why the mass extinction took place. But fossil records show a die-off of several species occurring about 251 million years ago.

The most supported view right now is that there was a large eruption of volcanoes in Siberia, which could have spewed out enough lava to cover Russia. Every time a volcano erupts, they release many greenhouse gases. The eruption of such a large number of volcanoes drastically shifted the balance of elements in the air, meaning organisms nearby were asphyxiated from a lack of oxygen or poisoned by an excess of carbon dioxide in the blood.[56]

Is this the future we are destined for? Elon Musk has been questioned for his ruthless march outwards towards Mars, the next frontier. But in the future, he may be celebrated for starting humanity on this path. However, I completely understand those who challenge going to Mars whilst our planet needs its own TLC.

Our society has overseen such unprecedented destruction of the natural world in such a short time that we are beginning to force nature's hand. Scientists have even started referring to this stage in Earth's life as the Anthropocene, meaning the age of man. The Anthropocene takes over from the Holocene, an age that has overseen one of the most stable periods of weather known to occur on Earth.

The Holocene, which is thought to have started in the last 11,000 years, also coincidentally began alongside the birth of that first known farming community in Göbekli Tepe. Before we entered the Holocene, Earth had spent roughly two million years in a period of glacial fluctuations, referred to as the Pleistocene or Ice Age.

The Holocene was and still is the barometer that a stable climate should be measured against. Scientists around the globe are now considering the possibility that we have accidentally ended this period of calm due to the side effects of our industrial society and that the Anthropocene is now well underway.

For humans to have had such a significant impact on our planet in only the last 200 years that we now enter a new stage of Earth's life is worth pausing to think about.

---

56 Black, 2010

One of the most impacted parts of our ecosystem is also one of the most important elements; the air we breathe. We all know how serious this situation is.

This chapter will look at the current predicament of air both outside and inside the home. It will look at what we as individuals can do to build a better relationship with the air around us.

CLEAN AIR

It is estimated that 92 percent of the world's population lives in sub-optimal air conditions. Pollutants in the air are linked to an increase in degenerative brain diseases such as Alzheimer's and Parkinson's, as well as difficulties during pregnancy such as miscarriages or the increased chance of autism and asthma in newborn children.

Trouble starts to occur when pollution in the air gets stuck in our nose and lungs, causing inflammation, which can lead to respiratory problems over time. If these are left untreated, it can drastically increase the likelihood that you will suffer from a serious illness in your lifetime.[57]

Sin of Synthetics

In 1907 Leo Hendrik Baekeland, a Belgian scientist living in New York, USA, made a significant discovery that would change the fate of all life on Earth. Baekeland was trying to find an alternative to shellac—a natural wood resin finish created from the feces of the female lac bug in India and Thailand. Due to this

---

57   Beelen et al., 2014

unique source, it was difficult to scale up the production of shellac, leaving the market open for a competitor product capable of delivering a similar quality resin in a scalable way.

Baekeland's research uncovered that it was possible to produce a hard shapable material by controlling the pressure and temperature applied to phenol and formaldehyde (now a known carcinogen). Plastic was born.

In this chapter, I will not be talking about the use of plastics and how the invention has coincided with a monumental leap forward for our society. This chapter is about the air around us and how the level of plastic use in our society has also started to impact the quality of our air.

Every month, a new study shows the risk of microplastics getting into our food and water streams. But through a process called outgassing, our plastic products are also getting into our air. There is now a whole stream of products we use daily, consistently outgassing harmful chemicals into our homes. Anything from nail polish remover to frying pans and air fresheners has the potential to cause us harm. The air around us and in our homes has been invaded.

We might feel powerless to do much about the air outside of our homes, but when the problem occurs within our own four walls, we have a responsibility to minimize the risks to our health as much as possible.

You know that smell when you get something new. A new book, a new car, a new video game, a freshly painted room . . . whatever it may be. What you are smelling is the product outgassing.

Outgassing is the name for the slow release of gases into the air. Unfortunately, in the case of plastics (alongside many other modern products), the gases typically released are dangerous chemicals. This is still a new body of research but is a perfect example of how our human ingenuity has raced ahead of our health needs as humans.

Dangerous airborne chemicals are being inhaled daily by us and our pets . It is not just the products with a distinctive smell you have to be worried about either. Even plastic-based products with no smell might still be capable of releasing chemical gases, or what scientists call VOCs (volatile organic compounds).

VOCs risk both short and long-term health, and exposure can cause symptoms such as skin irritation, allergic response, sore throat, difficulty breathing, headaches and more.[58]

Let's take mattresses, for example. When I bought my first mattress, I remember having to choose between thickness, number of springs, and memory foam, among other features. However, not once did we consider the risk that the mattress we were buying would contaminate our home while it shed its gases. But why would we worry about that? After all, what company would create a product they knew would contaminate their customers' homes and not tell them?

But that is precisely what our new mattress would go on to do. Looking back, I was surprised by the strong smell it gave off upon opening. With hindsight, it is now obvious that as soon as I opened the mattress and rolled it out, it was simply starting the long process of outgassing any stored VOCs into the air.

How could I have avoided this outgassing problem? The worst outgassing occurs in the first few days, but I have seen recommendations advising that a new mattress is stored in a cross-ventilated

---

58 Poslusny, 2018

area for the first two weeks after opening.[59] Because we all have a cross-ventilated space to store a new mattress when we get it, right?

A Californian study published in Environmental Science & Technology in July 2019 looked at the release of VOCs during a typical night's sleep for an adult. The mattresses used in the study had been allowed to outgas for six months. The study showed that when body heat is released as infrared during the night, it increases the outgassing capabilities of the mattress, sending an increased amount of VOCs into the air when compared to the outgassing when the mattress was not in use.

For most people, this increased level of outgassing remained below the "No Significant Risk Levels" set by Californian environmental laws. But, if you take the results from the study and skew them to account for a young child's profile, the results are more concerning. Researchers showed that the outgassed cancer-causing compounds such as formaldehyde and benzene were close to or exceeded risk levels for young children.[60]

We tend to be more flippant with our health. But are we ever flippant with the health of our children?

This does not mean we have to throw away all products in our house that have been manufactured using chemicals. We would all have very little left. For me, it would mean getting rid of most of my flatpack furniture and other items made from pressed wood, along with my carpets and plastic kitchen furnishings, among many more. However, there are things we can do now without getting rid of anything.

---

59 Golde, 2022

60 Thompson, 2019

Outside air is clean air. Despite what we are doing to the climate, outside air can still be up to 10x less toxic than the air in our homes.

Improving the air quality in your home is as simple as opening a couple of windows. As a resident of central London, I used to believe that I should keep my windows closed to keep the toxicity of the city out and all the good air in. But I am collecting pollution inside as well, and I need to let it out from time to time. Every day I make sure that we have a couple of windows open, or at least on the latch, letting a blow-through of fresh air circulate.

Remember that whenever you bring something new into your home and do not know what it is made of, it may be worth giving time to outgas, to reduce the risk to you and your family's health.

I am sure that some companies out there are well aware of the damage caused by their products outgassing in people's homes and take every measure to minimize that risk. In cases like this, the responsible manufacturer can give their products time to outgas before they go to market. If you are ever concerned, I would recommend reaching out to the manufacturer of a product with a high risk of outgassing harmful VOCs a few weeks before purchase and asking if they will open the packing and let the product you are buying outgas before delivery.

There are other recommended ways to avoid exposure to VOCs inside your home. Buying used products is a great way to ensure you are purchasing a product that has had enough time to outgas the most dangerous chemicals. As well as having a lower impact on the environment. Furthermore, buying furniture made of solid wood instead of pressed wood is another great way to avoid unnecessary exposure to the chemicals required to bond pressed wood together.[61]

A simple sniff test can be used on products in the home to establish whether they are outgassing or not. If the object does not smell strongly, it may have already given off many of its chemicals. However, if there is a significant smell, especially from new products, it may be worth allowing this product to outgas in a safe environment.

Allowing products to outgas safely can be a lengthy process. It is possible to speed up the process by using sunlight. There are many benefits to sunlight, which is the topic of the next chapter, one of those being the ability for solar heat to outgas dangerous VOCs. It is as simple as placing any object that needs outgassing into a sunny spot and slowly rotating throughout the day to ensure all surfaces are exposed. After an afternoon in the sun, apply the sniff test again and, if necessary, repeat the experiment until the chemical "new product smell" has lessened.

Please be aware that sunlight also causes the color in some products to fade, so if that is a concern, only leave it outside for a few hours. Leaving sensitive items in a shaded area will still allow for the benefits, albeit reduced, but will protect the color from fading.

Plant Friends

Despite our best efforts, there will likely be VOCs in the air of many modern homes. As we already discussed, letting clean air circulate and ventilate is one effective way to clean the air in your

---

61 How Scared Should You Be of Off-Gassing?, 2015

home. Another way to clean the air in your home, plants! Our leafy friends have been organically cleaning the air on our planet since way before we came along, and they can be of use in the home too.

Much of the research in this field comes from the space sector, with NASA accredited with many breakthroughs in the air cleaning industry. The NASA Clean Air Study was created to research ways to clean space station air. The research started in the 1980s and began by exploring the impacts on air when organizations switched to more energy-efficient building design, improving insulation and reducing fresh air exchange. Businesses were being encouraged to switch to this more energy-efficient building style as a way of saving costs. However, there was no thought to the impact of reduced airflow.

Upon occupation of these new buildings, workers began complaining about health issues such as itchy eyes, skin rashes, drowsiness, and headaches. The study says that "man himself should be considered another source of indoor air pollution, especially when living in a closed, poorly ventilated area."

Sick building syndrome is the name given to buildings suffering from poor airflow. WHO estimates that 30 percent of new buildings in the western world were suffering from varying degrees of air pollution at the time of the study.

NASA believed that beyond reducing the outgassing of equipment, they could also use plants and their associated soil micro-organisms to support the clean-up. The study contains many poignant anecdotes saying that "man's existence on Earth depends upon a life support system involving an intricate relationship with plants and their associated microorganisms; it should be obvious that when he attempts to isolate himself in tightly sealed buildings away from this ecological system, problems will arise."

What an excellent assessment of our relationship with planet Earth. Imagine if we applied that line of thinking when developing all technology.

NASA goes on to say that if our society is to move into a closed environment on Earth or in space, they will need to find a way to bring nature's life support system with them. The starting point for this research has evolved from a body of work looking at wastewater treatment where plants have been used alongside an activated carbon filter to remove toxic components.

The air is filtered through an activated carbon filter where VOCs are absorbed. Plant roots and other microorganisms destroy any dangerous viruses, bacteria, or organic chemicals, eventually converting these air pollutants into new plants. Chemicals used during the study include benzene and formaldehyde, two of the most common dangerous chemicals we typically find outgassed by synthetic material.

A wide variety of plants were used in the study, ranging from bamboo palm to English ivy and serpents tongue to peace lily. The results showed us that different plants are better at removing different chemicals. For example, if you wanted a plant to remove the chemical benzene from the air, there was one clear winner. At over 100,000 micrograms removed per plant, the gerbera daisy is the clear front runner with the second-best air cleaner, the pot mum plant, only managing 76,000 micrograms removed per plant.

However, if you wanted to remove formaldehyde from the air, you would be better off going for serpents tongue, which could remove over 31,000 micrograms of the pollutant despite the leaves only having a surface area of 2,800 cm2. Another solid performer was the bamboo palm, which removed 76,000 micrograms of formaldehyde, although this required a much larger surface leafage of almost 14,500 cm2.[62]

The study summarizes that low-light requiring houseplants, along with activated carbon filters, have the potential for substantially improving air quality in an enclosed space by removing pollutants. They believe that the plant system is the most effective way of treating sick building syndrome and that the plant root-soil zone is the most effective area for removing VOCs.

So, grow plants in big pots if possible. They will make your air cleaner. Amber and I keep lots of plants, and we make sure to keep plenty of the best air cleaners, serpents tongue and peace lily, in our bedroom for healthy clean air.

One disturbing trend I see, that counteracts the act of buying plants for air condition, are all the fake plastic plants entering the market. Not only are fake plants unable to keep the air around us clean, but they are also bringing in another pollutant that may be causing damage to our health over the long term.

AIRBATHING

There is no wonder that humans feel improved well-being after time in nature. It is one of the few times that we are breathing air similar to the air that our ancestors breathed 11,000 years ago.

Green Cities

A study that moved 110 children from a high air pollution area to a low air pollution area and monitored them over ten years,

---

62 Wolverton, Johnson and Bounds, 1989

showed that their lungs improved in performance and comparative growth. And not only did their lungs perform better, but they developed more effectively too.[63]

This is the price we pay for city life. I must admit that when I moved to London in 2016, I was not aware of the severity of the problem. Like everyone, I assumed it was not good to breathe polluted air. But I felt that if the issue were so severe, it would be more of a news topic.

In London, scientists performed a study on people with either a clean bill of health or a history of lung/heart disease. Participants of the study were randomly assigned a 2-hour walk along either Oxford Street (one of the busiest high streets in England) or Hyde Park (an ample green space neighboring Oxford Street). This research, which the British Heart Foundation funded, interpreted that those walking on Oxford Street with increased exposure to air pollution had the forced vital capacity of your lungs impacted, or the amount of air you can exhale after a large inhalation.

However, the participants who were asked to walk through Hyde Park experienced the opposite, as they experienced an increase in their lung capacity in the hours after their walk.[64]

Anyone who has spent time in London has most likely travelled there due to its status as one of the major cities in our society. London is a mecca for many people, whether for work or leisure. However, the chances are small that somebody would travel to London just for its green spaces.

---

63 AVOL et al., 2001
64 Sinharay et al., 2018

Despite that being the case, it is still one of the greenest cities in the world, and although it has not quite achieved the utopian vision of becoming a "national park city," it is well on the way, with 18 percent of London currently comprised of green space.

Compare that to the 13 percent in Toronto and an even greater 27 percent in New York, and it is clear that modern cities are giving attention to green spaces.

On the other side of the globe, the city of Singapore is located on an island just south of Malaysia. With much of the significant developments of the city coming well into the late 20th century, designers could capitalize on the catalogue of learnings provided by the development of all other cities up to that point.

In the same way, cities like Barcelona, New York and San Francisco were built in a grid system to make them easier to navigate. Singapore is now being built organically, with access to nature and green spaces a defining feature of the environment. The city of Singapore currently has a massive 47 percent green coverage, with aims to continue down the road of becoming the world's greenest city. Or the garden city, as they like it to be called.

However, despite all of this work to build a more organic city, Singapore is still struggling with a major air pollution problem. It seems that no amount of greenery can sequester the island city's emissions.

With two-thirds of the world's population (currently that would mean five billion people) estimated to be living in cities by 2050, maybe we need to start thinking about the solutions to this problem right now.

Singapore is trying to clean up its act. It became the first Southeast Asian city to join the BreatheLife campaign. The

BreatheLife campaign was jointly launched by WHO, UN Environment and the Climate and Clean Air Coalition.

Their primary objective is to reduce the number of deaths related to air pollution by 2030 and slow the rate of climate change. To do this, the campaign is delivering projects across various areas such as walking and cycling networks, wastewater treatment, passive building design (more on that later), emission standards and mass transport systems. For the first time in my life, we are seeing a global movement focused on improving air quality accessible on a city level instead of a country level.

The cities of the future will be shaped by their responsibility to keep our air clean. Up to this point, and for some time more, the residents of cities will have to continue suffering from sub-optimal air quality and the health impacts it brings.

Whether it is the switch from coal to cleaner energy sources in some of the worst polluted cities in the world or the continued reduction of cars in some of the world's cleanest cities, the fight is on to create safe havens where high numbers of humans can work, live and play together without putting their health or their family's health at risk.

Forest Bathing

Regardless of what we know, there is so much we still do not know about the fragile ecosystem we are a part of. Until we get to the point where we have all the answers, we must ensure that we protect the wide variety of life around us as we all evolve alongside each other and right now, we still rely on each other as we continue evolving.

It is not just the cleanliness of the natural air that improves our well-being. Forest air contains phytoncides, airborne chemical compounds that protect trees and other plants from bacterial, fungal and insect attacks. They operate in the air similarly to VOCs. However, they provide beneficial rather than harmful effects on our health.

One study looked at the health benefits of spending time in the widespread bamboo forests in Southwestern China. Sixty male participants were split between spending three days in a bamboo forest and three days in urban environments. Blood pressure, heart rate and oxygen saturation were measured as markers of physical health, and a mood state questionnaire was used to measure mental health.

Results showed that time spent in a bamboo forest enhanced positive mood states and reduced negative ones. Blood pressure and heart rate also decreased, whilst oxygen saturation increased. Bamboo forest therapy also increased the number of Natural Killer (NK) cells in the participants.[65] NK cells are cancer-fighting proteins that seek and destroy any tumor and virus-ridden cells.

Other studies have corroborated similar benefits of spending time in nature, with a study of forty-eight Japanese males concluding that walking in a forest may promote cardiovascular relaxation and reduce negative psychological symptoms.[66]

Forests can be used to help improve both physical and mental health. We can rewild our well-being simply by spending time in these green spaces. Every time we step into the woods, we have a

65   Lyu et al., 2019

66   Lee et al., 2014

chance to reconnect to nature in the same way our ancestors lived and thrived.

We have evolved to spend time in these places regardless of weather, with extra benefits to our health found during and after rainfall.

Petrichor is the earthy scent produced when rain falls on dry soil. Maybe we enjoy the smell of nature during rainfall because of the oils, pollen and fungal spores released into the air, which we then inhale into our lungs.

Specifically, the pleasant smell comes from soil microbes such as *Streptomyces* releasing the molecule *geosmin*. This earthy scent can then be breathed into our lungs alongside countless other bacteria, fungal spores and pollen to contribute to a healthy lung biome.

We are still in the early days of exploring what we know about these tiny helpers, but technology is opening doors to new ways of researching them every day. Each year, we learn a little bit more about how closely the fate of our health is tied to the fate of the unique biome in our body.

As a species of animal that evolved from a playground of trees and wildlife, it makes sense that we may have a deep symbiosis with the natural world. Our ancestors have been exposed to these environments for millions of years. If we follow Darwinism, it makes sense that the mere practice of evolution would favor those individuals that found a way to get a health benefit from the forest air surrounding them.

Unfortunately, most of us do not have the luxury of living in an old-growth forest's lush environment. More likely, we are living in modern homes, built with modern building methods and surrounded by various modern devices.

But we can all spend more time in nature to get the benefits. Every time you spend time in a green space with trees, you choose to support your lung microbiome, improving your health and well-being.

To fully immerse in the airbathing experience is to break down the barriers between you and the natural world. The more time we spend in nature, the more resilient our bodies become.

A quick and easy way to clock up lots of airbathing time is to go on a camping trip. Regardless of your level of comfort in nature, we can all find a trip that allows us to sleep with the fresh air of nature around us. Amber and I do this by wild camping in forests and mountains and by staying in pods and yurts.

In the Seven Practices Challenge, we challenge people to spend an entire day outside. When was the last time you tried that? You can take the Challenge yourself by going to www.beyond-domestication.com.

ACTIVE BREATHING

I remember reading the Seven Habits of Highly Effective People by Steven Covey in 2015. In a chapter discussing Maslow's hierarchy of needs, he asks the reader to think about what they desire most in life. At that point in my life, my brain was thinking about health, career progression and money. However, Covey followed that question by saying, "Imagine if I took all of the oxygen out of the room or car you are in right now; what would your lead desire be then?"

That one got me. I had never considered that out of everything in life, my base desire was and still is for oxygen (and then plenty of other essentials like water and food) long before I thought about money or my career.

For something so important, our society takes it for granted. I am not just talking about the air we breathe but how we breathe. For most of us, breathing is an unconscious task completed by our subconscious 24 hours a day, 365 days a year.

Yet despite all of the challenges we face in our lives, there is no one point where you have managed to go without oxygen for anything more than short periods (the world record for longest breath-hold is over 22 minutes, set by Stig Severinsen, but that is only possible by breathing pure oxygen from a tank during preparation).

Breathwork

The use of breath for well-being is not new science; in some circles, it has been around for years. Practices like yoga already promote active breathwork, with specific forms of yoga such as pranayama focusing specifically on the breath rather than the physicality.

We can all take back control of this primal behavior from our subconscious. Breath can be used as a tool for recovery and self-learning, with a myriad of benefits coming from a rediscovery of active breathing.

The first step to understanding your breath is exploring your pattern of breathing. As you grow older and more detached from active breathwork, you may use less of your respiratory system.

Personally, at the start of my reconnection to the practice of air, I was a deep chest breather and would watch my chest muscles moving slowly up and down with each breath. In contrast, if you watch a newborn baby sleeping, they breathe into both their chest and their belly, or more specifically, their diaphragm. We all breathe differently, and active breathing is about unlocking the part of the respiratory system that can lay dormant for us.

As someone who has been a long-term chest breather, or shallow breather as it is more commonly known, I have not taken full advantage of my lung capacity. As a shallow breather, when taking a breath, I could only draw in a minimal amount of air into my lungs each time. And despite minimal air being enough to get the job done, there are still consequences for not breathing to our total capacity. Instead, I could have been breathing into my belly, using the full range of my diaphragm.

Scientists have proven that when only drawing in a minimal amount of air and not using the muscles in your diaphragm to breathe, you are at increased risk of various anxiety disorders, including stress and panic attacks.[67]

It was surprising to me that something as simple as our breath can have such a big impact on something as significant as our mood, but that is precisely the case. How we breathe directly affects the way we live, and we can use it as a tool to impact our moods.

One of the easiest and thus my favorite methods of active breathing is the simple 5-second exhale. We all build up stressors in our life, and for those times when everything starts to feel overwhelming and out of your control, a simple inhale and 5-second exhale may hold the answer. This is because breathing out for 5 seconds triggers a command to tell your central nervous system to relax.

---

67   Zaccaro et al., 2018

It is believed that our ability as humans to use our breath this way is a hangover from our time spent hunting in the wild. In the context of our wild ancestors, it would only have been possible to pause and exhale for 5 seconds if they were in a place of total safety, and that is what we are tapping into now.

When we give ourselves the time to exhale over 5 seconds slowly, we are telling our body that we are in a safe place, instantly triggering a sense of relaxation throughout our central nervous system. Again, this might not seem like a groundbreaking solution. But I can guarantee that this will calm you down almost instantly. The next time you feel that red mist rising, stop, slow down and breathe.

The first time I tried this technique was after being offered redundancy by my workplace. After the initial panic and shock, on the phone to Amber she reminded me to stop and breathe. After taking the time to breathe in for five seconds and out for five seconds, my anxiety about the future washed away, and my mind cleared.

I remember that moment for the euphoria of positively experiencing active breathing rather than the difficulty of facing redundancy. It is one of my earliest memories from my rewilding journey.

Active breathwork is also used as a treatment for people addicted to smoking. One theory suggests that a large part of the desire to smoke is just the desire to breathe actively. Even though nicotine may play a part, relaxation comes from the deep inhale and the long, smooth exhale.

To test this, dependent smokers were asked to take a 4-hour break from smoking. During this time, they partook in controlled deep breathing every 30 minutes, sitting quietly between these breathing sessions.

Miraculously, all the participants of this study found their cravings easier to manage. What the scientists discovered is that it was possible to use active breathing as a method of fighting cigarette withdrawals. Not only that, but the participants still felt the positive benefits of smoking, mentioning that they still felt awake and able to concentrate as if they had just had a cigarette.[68]

Mindful Breathing

Using your breath to calm stressors in your life and as a way of quitting smoking is already a pretty profound reason to take active breathwork seriously. But one man has taken it to a completely different level, using the breath to perform feats once thought impossible by the world of science. He has even shown his body to be capable of fighting off severe bacterial infections such as e-coli by using breathwork to boost his immune system.

The man is, of course, Wim Hof. Mentioned in the last chapter for his love of cold water therapy, the Iceman—as he has become known, has been marveling the world of science since he first started breaking world records in 2000.

The experiment I mentioned above is a real one. It is no joke that he willingly submitted himself to being injected with live e-coli bacterium to prove to the scientific world that he could influence his autonomic nervous system, a feat once thought impossible. Even the word autonomic (which describes the

---

68 McClernon, Westman and Rose, 2004

nervous system he influenced) is defined in the dictionary as either involuntary or unconscious.

The results obtained by the Radboud University Nijmegen Medical Centre in 2011 were nothing short of remarkable, as Wim provided the scientists with categoric evidence of the control he has over his immune response. To achieve this, after being injected with e-coli, Wim used his practice of breathwork and meditation to enable the increase in his level of the stress hormone, cortisol.

Cortisol is used by the body to suppress the immune response, and in Wim's case, his increased levels meant that he had an immune response over 50 percent lower than the expected baseline.[69]

Considering that e-coli harms the body by tricking your immune cells into attacking itself, Wim's solution of reducing his immune response completely negated all typical side effects and allowed him a full recovery.

Understandably, in the case of a single point of evidence, the term "the exception proves the rule" is usually applied, and in this case, Wim was undoubtedly the exception.

However, Wim did not stop there. He was highly confident of his ability to train others in the same practices he uses to alter his immune response, so a follow-up study was born. For the follow-up, 24 brave individuals also volunteered to be injected

---

69 Research on 'Iceman' Wim Hof suggests it may be possible to influence autonomic nervous system and immune response, 2011

with the e-coli endotoxin. 12 of the 24 individuals joined Wim in Poland for a period of training, including active breathwork and cold water exposure, and the remaining 12 were used as the control group. I can only imagine how the control group felt going into the experiment!

As you may expect, the individuals that trained with Wim were capable of boosting their cortisol levels to the point where on average, they experienced fewer flu-like symptoms than the candidates with no prior training.

Matthijs Kox, the author of the first study and one of the scientists performing these studies at Radboud University, suspects that Wim's breathing technique is the most significant contributor to the reduced immune response shown by the study participants. Even in the 30 minutes before the e-coli had been injected, Wim's trained group's active breathwork showed them to produce more adrenaline as their immune systems readied their defenses.

The scientists in Holland now aim to isolate the specific impact of the breathing exercise and replicate this study with more volunteers.[70]

Our breath holds the key to a different way of experiencing life. We can control the level of oxygen inside us, just as we control the amount of water we drink, and as humans, we can use it as a tool to support well-being.

I spoke to buteyko breath coach Kevin O'Neill, also known as Breatheolution. Kev is an Oxygen Advantage instructor and has been an inspiration of mine as he was the first person to coach me into the cold with my breath on the Unguarded Warrior retreat.

---

70   Kox et al., 2014

Kev said that people are generally over breathing, which affects biochemistry and mental health. This habit of breathing quicker than recommended is also, in some cases, leading to symptoms of chronic hyperventilation.

He told me that the recommended time for an inhale and exhale should be about five to five and a half seconds each, which may be much more than you think! Over 10 seconds to complete one inhale and exhale.

He also explained the impact of shallow breathing, where people are not utilizing the full range of their diaphragm result in a loss of up to 18 percent of potential oxygen intake per breath. This failure to adequately fill the lungs can lead to anxiety and vulnerability in places you may have used to feel comfortable.

Kev went on to tell me that as mammals, we should be using our noses to breathe. The mouth contains no functions to support healthy breath; it is all connected to food. Whereas, if you look at the nose, it is designed intricately to process the air coming in and out of our lungs.

I have experienced a journey with nasal breathing, and I now opt to breathe predominantly through my nose during exercise. This limited my ability to perform specific cardio at first but only until my ability to breathe nasally had increased over time.

Take the advice from Kev with you from this chapter. Breathe through your nose and slow it down. Five seconds in, five seconds out. Think about how amazing it is that your body has evolved to use the oxygen in the air around you as fuel for your body and that without it, life as we know it would end.

Seven Practice Recommendations

- Shop second hand
- Open your windows daily
- Grow air-cleaning plants (serpent tongue and peace lily)
- Spend time forest bathing
- Breathe actively through your nose
- Breathe outside every day
- Camp overnight in nature

PRACTICE 4

SUNLIGHT

FOR YEARS, OUR society has put the Earth firmly at the center of the universe, with all the stars and planets spinning perfectly around us. They were a part of our story, and we played the leading role.

That is the story our society has fostered for longer than it has known the truth. And how the truth changed everything. In our current understanding of Earth and space, we are not the stars of the show. We are not even supporting actors. Despite the delicate alignment of so many variables that, over time, has protected the fragile balance of life on Earth through its evolution. On the scale of the universe, we are nothing.

We looked at how we interact with the food, water, and air in our landscape, and now we need to look at how we interact with the sun. For 4.5 billion years, our sun has burned, using its vast gravitational pull to contain itself—and the rest of our solar system. The sun is the real star of our show, and once its time in the limelight is up (in around five billion years), life on Earth will end with it.

To get us into the mindset for sunlight, I want us to think again about our practice of air. We know that when we breathe, we input oxygen as fuel and exhale waste air as carbon dioxide. Pretty simple to understand. Even though it occurs off the visible spectrum, we have all been taught to understand how our lungs utilize the oxygen in the air.

A very similar thing happens every time we go out into the sun. Our body harnesses beneficial nutrients whenever we are exposed to natural light. Just like we cannot see the oxygen in the air being converted to carbon dioxide as we walk around, we also do not see our exchange of nutrients with the sun, but we can feel it.

Spectrums of Light

The sun is the real star of our show, and light is one of the byproducts created by the sun as it gives off electromagnetic radiation into space. This sunlight, which has to make the long journey from the sun to the Earth, is made up of visible, ultraviolet and infrared energy.

Once it has travelled the 8.3-minute journey from the sun to Earth, it is filtered through our atmosphere to become the sunlight that makes everything on Earth just that little bit brighter . . . The part of sunlight responsible for brightening up our planet is visible light, the portion of sunlight visible to the naked eye. A rainbow is a perfect example of the visible light spectrum.

Ultraviolet light has a shorter frequency than visible light, making it invisible to the naked eye. Responsible for many a tan line, ultraviolet light is also capable of damaging our DNA as well as sterilizing any surfaces that it comes into contact with. However, within the dangers of ultraviolet light hides vitamin D.

Vitamin D is unique among vitamins in its ability to be absorbed by human skin from contact with sunlight alone. According to the NHS England website, vitamin D is responsible for regulating the amount of calcium and phosphate in the body, with a deficiency in vitamin D potentially leading to bone deformities such as rickets in children and bone pain in adults.[71] Understanding vitamin D in our body is one of the simplest health benefits we can control.

A natural way to manage your vitamin D is to take more active control of your sunlight exposure. You can support your body's health by directly considering the impact of exposing or not exposing yourself to sunlight and the duration you should be exposing yourself.

Infrared light is another form of light not visible to the human eye. We detect it simply in the form of heat. As humans, we absorb the infrared heat from the sun and then slowly radiate it off. In the same way, the sun can be said to be giving off radiation, so are we.

If you walk into a room full of people with the lights on, you can look around and see everyone. However, as soon as the lights are turned off, everybody will fade into the darkness. Infrared light operates on a completely different part of the spectrum, separate from the visible light that we can see. Through infrared goggles, human bodies would reappear as little radiators. Balls of warmth among the cooler ambient temperature of the room.

Human bodies are constantly adapting in response to the different light given off by our sun. Over years of evolution, this has helped shape humanity into the diversity of races we now see across the globe.

---

71 Overview - Rickets and osteomalacia

WHERE ARE WE FROM?

Homo sapiens have travelled a long way in the last 50,000–70,000 years. Before the birth of our current society, our ancient ancestors had already explored much of the globe, traversing what are now massive oceanic bodies of water.

These ice ages led to vastly higher quantities of water being stored as ice near the poles, which drastically lowered the global sea level. The lower sea level allowed humans of the time to simply walk out of East Africa into much of Asia and Oceania, even making it from the tip of Southern Asia into what we now call Australia—all without boats.

Natural Selection

Early humans also took advantage of a similar opportunity when it presented itself to reach what we now call America. In contrast to the humans crossing into Australia by walking across the sea floor, early Homo sapiens were able to cross into America over what is known as the Bering land bridge, the passage of water between Russia and Alaska. When the weather was cold enough for it to freeze, it was possible to walk freely between Europe and America.

Changing weather led to the melting of the Bering land bridge, which subsequently increased sea levels. This change in weather isolated communities of Homo sapiens across not just America but multiple islands, albeit some islands that were the size of continents.

Everywhere that humanity spread, they have faced slightly different levels of sunlight, providing the catalyst for all the different races within the species of Homo sapiens that we see today.

Scientists have a theory that as Homo sapiens began to lose their hair in exchange for sweat glands, they naturally became more vulnerable to harmful ultraviolet light leading to the change in skin color that we see today. Changing skin color occurred due to the evolution of melanin. Melanin occurs naturally in the body in varying amounts as a way of absorbing and dispersing ultraviolet light from your surroundings.

It is believed that as exposure to the ultraviolet levels in sunlight changed, the melanin levels in our skin pigmentation were affected. As we travelled further north, the days started to get shorter, and the sun's angle started to get lower in the sky. The further from the equator we travelled, the fairer our skin became, enabling us to produce adequate amounts of vitamin D during the summer to take us through the long winter months, when the sun is no longer giving off vitamin D.[72]

Worldwide Experiments

For the last 500 years, we have been conducting several worldwide experiments.

Since the first long-distance journeys were made by boat, vast numbers of humans have been able to settle in previously inaccessible areas. Locations such as Australia have now become the home for millions of humans who are more naturally adapted for a lifetime spent further away from the equator.

---

72 Jablonski, 2013

If we look at the recent colonization of Australia and New Zealand throughout the 1800s, it is clear that the skin of the locals contrast with that of the settlers. Unique in its own way, the aboriginals of Australia were able to develop their pigmentation over the 50,000 years since they left East Africa.

What risk did the early settlers of Australia and all subsequent non-native settlers run by living outside of their natural environment?

Since this colonization of Australia, citizens have gone on to develop the highest instances of melanoma and other skin cancers, with people of fairer skin significantly affected. Aboriginal groups are also affected but in much smaller numbers.

Between 2005–2009, the rate of melanoma in Indigenous Australians was 9.3 cases per 100,000 people, compared to 33 cases per 100,000 in non-native Australians.[73] Put simply, the adapted indigenous skin-type makes you three times less likely to be at risk of melanoma and other skin cancer than Australians with fairer skin.

SAFE SUNBATHING

I feel like the keyword for sunlight is safety. Despite inviting people to spend time outdoors in sunlight to boost both mental and physical health and well-being, it may not be entirely safe for us to go from living indoors for 90 percent of our day to spending 90 percent outdoors.

---

73   Sima, 2016

It is a fact that the sun is trying to kill us (not that I imagine this is a personal vendetta) and that only protection from the Earth's atmosphere stops us from being fried by radiation.

Vitamin D

With my skin tone, if I were living in Australia, I would want to manage my time in the sun carefully—a day spent tanning without consideration or protection would be unlikely!

Our bodies require vitamin D to operate effectively, and our varying melanin levels have evolved to allow us to expose ourselves to natural vitamin D as safely as possible. We can see the impact of this in America, where there is a notably higher vitamin D deficiency among African Americans compared to other Americans.[74]

America and other countries along a similar latitude have less access to natural vitamin D than countries closer to the equator. The further north you travel, the less vitamin D is available from the sun throughout the year.

Going into winter, as the sun's angle becomes lower in the sky, there can be many months where the sun is too low for ultraviolet light to pierce through the Earth's atmosphere, reducing the risk from any harmful rays and access to the beneficial rays as well.

The lower the angle the sunlight hits the Earth, the more atmosphere it has to pass through, effectively filtering out the beneficial rays before they can reach the surface. Cities in a similar latitude to London, New York, Berlin and Paris only get access

---

74 Harris, 2006

to natural vitamin D between March and October, with the sun remaining below 30 degrees in the sky during the winter months.

In some cases, science recommends supplementation as the best way to receive extra vitamin D. While I would not usually support this avenue, giving your body a helping hand can be necessary if the sun is not there to do it for you.

You can also supplement by eating whole foods like salmon, eggs and mushrooms that contain more natural forms of vitamin D.

We are just beginning to understand the nuanced benefits of exposure to natural sunlight. We now know that sunlight can trigger the release of serotonin and endorphins while reducing the risk of prostate, breast, and pancreatic cancers. It can reduce inflammation and improve our circadian rhythms. And the icing on the cake is that it improves virtually every mental condition you can think of. All for free.[75]

We do not understand all of the gifts that the sun gives us, and until we do, we will have to make time in our routine for a practice of regular, safe sun exposure.

What we have witnessed over the last 11,000 years and are still witnessing today is the slow retreat by our society to the creature comforts of the indoors. No longer are we our ancient ancestors who lived predominantly under the sky and the stars.

Back in 2001, a study published in Nature commented that Americans already spent 93 percent of their time indoors or only 1 hour and 40 minutes outside.[76] I wonder what that looks like today?

_____

75   Murray, 2013
76   Klepeis et al., 2001

We are elite builders, creating many spaces with the remit of keeping nature out and fighting against it rather than with it. The advice is clear, and the risks are real. With sunlight deficiency continuing to lead to ill health, it may be time for us to reevaluate how and where we live, work and play.

I picture a world where we are not just chasing a suntan during a summer holiday to warmer climates but also regularly expose ourselves to natural sunlight where we live. If you can make time for regular sunlight as part of your daily routine, you can rack up plenty of safe sunbathing hours and feel healthier.

These decisions do not have to be groundbreaking. Opting for the beer garden at the pub rather than sitting inside, standing on the platform at the train station rather than sitting in the waiting room or going for a road run rather than using a treadmill. There are many ways to reengage with our ancient physiology, and time spent outside will help us along this journey.

With many of us adapting to hybrid working, what about taking your desk outside for that sneaky safe sun exposure during the workday? Even if you sit in the shade, you will still benefit from time in nature.

Is there a spot in your garden, balcony, or local park where you can take advantage of a sunny day by working outside for a few hours?

When we do safely sunbathe, it is imperative we give vitamin D and the other benefits time to soak into the skin. When you expose yourself to the sun, treat your skin gently after. Let it enjoy all the benefits that the sun brings naturally.

One tool I use to help me with my safe sunbathing is the smartphone app dminder. The app considers skin type, location, sun angle, clothing, age, and body type to track your natural vitamin D exposure and recommend safe limits for unprotected sun time.

I use the app to help understand how potent the sun is on each day and use it to know when to either cover up or leave the sunlight. Always trust your body before the app. If you are going red, cover up or get inside.

The data dminder presents helped me to learn more about the potency of the sun in different locations and how it impacts me personally.

Eyesight

We are not powerless in our defense from the sun. One method of sun protection that has become particularly popular in our society is sunglasses.

Worn by many for fashion (or nursing a hangover), sunglasses have become one of the most iconic accessories. Considered a fashion item, they are worn by many of us whenever we get the opportunity. Only a tiny bit of sun? No problem, time for the shades.

However, whenever we put on sunglasses, we put up a barrier to the natural world, preventing nature from running its course. As we will see shortly, 80 percent of young adults in Singapore developed myopia from a lack of exposure to sunlight and items like sunglasses make it harder to take advantage of the benefits of sunlight.[77]

A study by the Sleep Medical Clinic proved that when sunlight reaches our eyes, it impacts little photoreceptors, helping to

---

77 Chia, 2021

set the body's circadian rhythm and improving sleep, mood, and appetite.[78] This is interrupted whenever we put glass between our eyes and the sun.

Of course, this is a balance, and sunglasses can still be a part of sun defense when used appropriately. When Doug Bock Clark, author of The Last Whalers, spent three years living with the Lamaleran tribe in South Thailand, he discovered a group of people that still live off the land, similarly to how their ancient ancestors would have subsisted. However, they also utilize modern conveniences like sunglasses to maintain their eyes' health.

Lamalerans are primarily subsisting off the local whale population, with spotters high up on the hills responsible for reporting whale water plumes to the rest of the village. Over time, the constant work of looking at the water, with the bright light of the sun reflecting straight off the surface into their eyes, leads to the whale spotters developing cataracts.

However, wearing sunglasses every time they watch for whales has made it possible to protect their eyes, simultaneously protecting their essential role in the community. A perfect example of striking the right balance with technology.

It is not just indigenous communities considering their relationship with safe sunbathing. In recent years there have been attempts worldwide to try and remedy exposure to vitamin D for our younger generations.

Both China and Singapore have trialed solutions with varying degrees of success. In China, they took it as far as building glass classrooms, although this unsurprisingly led to a greenhouse effect more suitable for tropical plants than children.

---

78 Duffy and Czeisler, 2009

Singapore, on the other hand, has tried a different approach, providing smartwatches to children that track how much exposure to sunlight each child is getting. Interestingly, Singapore did not try this to reduce the number of threatening health conditions caused by a lack of vitamin D, but rather as a way of stemming the increased levels of myopia their younger generations are suffering from.

Myopia (short-sighted) is the most common diagnosis of impaired vision for people under 40. The main symptom is an increased difficulty in seeing distant objects clearly, ultimately hampering someone's ability to engage with the world around them as entirely as possible.

In 2010, an estimated 1.9 billion people worldwide were myopic,[79] with most cases developing in childhood. This makes the findings from the childhood study in Singapore even more crucial. Could they hold the key to understanding and potentially reducing the rising impact of myopia on our society's youth?

With 80 percent of young adults in Singapore currently diagnosed as short-sighted, the situation is growing ever more severe.

Singapore is on the cusp of a generation that may have difficulty seeing simple things like road signs or films at the cinema. The ramifications of this could end up forcing the government in Singapore to revolutionize their public spaces, including their travel networks, to support the large group of their populace who may become unable to clearly see objects located further away.

Professor Saw Seang Mai is the head of myopia research at the Singapore Eye Research Institute and the pioneer of the

---

79   Fricke et al., 2018

smartwatch project. Sensibly, Mai and her team are trying to get ahead of this right now, believing that sunlight holds the answer.

Two years before the smartwatch trial, they had experimented with measuring light intensities (lux) in different conditions. What they found was that, on a sunny day, light intensity outdoors can reach 100,000 lux and higher. However, when they repeated the same test indoors, they could only measure about 200–500 lux. A potential 200 times reduction in light intensity from spending time indoors instead of outside.

Mai hypothesized that this could be why time spent in sunlight is considered part of the cure for Singapore's growing myopia epidemic.

The increased light intensity outdoors can encourage the body to produce dopamine, which in the case of myopia, can support the growth of the eye during childhood. This prevents the eyeball from elongating during its development, which is the underlying cause of myopia.

The smartphone trial was considered a success not only because of the information gathered during the study but also because of the education it provided the children. Children were put against each other on a leaderboard, encouraging competition to see who could spend the most time outside.

Good performers were awarded gold badges on the app, with the best performers awarded a platinum badge. A parent of two of the children in the study said they are now "far more aware that they need to spend time outside. There is healthy competition. Once you have a community to compare with or if there are leaderboards online, that also helps."[80]

---

80 Bei Yi, 2015

CLIMATE

Since the first life forms were conceived, the sun has been a constant figure in daily Earth life. However, the negative impact of this heating system is growing on a global scale.

Like infrared heating devices, the sun works by heating the planet through thermal waves, not heating the air but the surfaces. We are now facing unprecedented warming as an increased amount of infrared radiation that used to come into contact with the surface of the Earth and then reflect safely back into space is now being trapped by the additional greenhouse gases we have added to our atmosphere.

Earth has had a natural greenhouse effect for as long as we have been evolving, and without it, Earth's surface would, on average, be 33°C cooler. By adding to the presence of greenhouse gases surrounding the Earth, we risk compromising delicate processes that have been operating for millennia.

Niche environments are currently most at risk, with glaciers, coral reefs and cloud forests (forests high in the mountains) being some of the most affected areas.[81]

We witnessed the first glacial casualty in 2019 when Okjökull in Iceland lost its fight against climate change.

As the first of 400 glaciers in Iceland to completely disappear, it was marked with a plaque containing a message to the future: "In the next 200 years, all our glaciers are expected to follow the same path. This monument is to acknowledge that we know what is happening and what needs to be done. Only you know if we did it."

---

81 Nunez, 2019

A somber message for a somber time. I hope that in 200 years, we can look back with thanks that we took the right path as a society.

Photosynthesis

One thing that has always amazed me is how plants photosynthesize sunlight into energy.

Plants use photosynthesis to turn energy from the sun into sugar and oxygen. Whereas animals like us need food, water, air, and sunlight to survive, plants can get by with just the last three. That simple process may hold one of the secrets to organic energy production.

At this point, we are not entirely useless at turning sunlight into energy. We have already been using solar panels for electricity, all the way back to those old-school desk calculators. Nowadays, solar panels are used on both an industrial and personal level, with massive solar farms and independent solar panels growing hugely in popularity since the beginning of the 21st century. However, this is not an organic approach to energy production. The development of solar panels has a finite lifetime; the precious metals used in production, like silver, are unsustainable. Furthermore, they perform poorly in low light conditions and storing any excess energy produced can be a struggle.

The evolution of plants is a popular avenue for science as it may hold the secrets to help us better understand the pathway towards organic energy production. One day, we may understand enough about that process that we can piggyback on the behavior of plants and produce our own clean energy. This is not a new idea; scientists worldwide are clamoring to be the first group to crack the code.

The potential for us to change the world is almost impossible to quantify. If we can find a way to produce energy using organic methods of power, then it may become possible to provide power to any part of the world where there is water, air, and sunlight.

One of the teams looking to tackle this issue is led by Boston College professor Dunwei Wang. His team has been trying to mimic photosynthesis and believes they may have reached a breakthrough in finding the formula.

The form of photosynthesis that Wang and his team have developed operates slightly differently from the traditional photosynthesis performed by plants. Unlike plants that only require sunlight, Wang and his colleagues used additional organic inputs to mimic plant photosynthesis. Using water and carbon dioxide combined with sunlight, they have found a way to produce energy that can be used to either fuel devices or be stored for consumption at a later date.[82]

Breakthroughs like this are fantastic news for the planet. If we can keep walking this path and find a way to bring a global solution to market, the potential for recovery of Earth's health will be greatly increased.

Wilderness Teacher

Every acre of wilderness that we have lost (and are still losing) may have been the key to one of humanity's present or future problems. As the only species capable of operating on a global

---

82 Zhao et al., 2018

scale, our society has developed a righteous existence, taking what we can for our gain, even when that means taking away from another human.

However, as the only global society, we are responsible for nurturing the planet that has birthed us, respecting all the wonderful lifeforms it has created. If rewilding is the answer, then Earth is the teacher, and as with all good subjects, we should pay attention and seek to learn whilst we still can.

This is not a job for just you or me. But a job for every member of our society. With the correct stories, people might be able to improve their understanding of the different lifeforms that populate our home with us, hopefully continuing to change the belief that we are unique and that this Earth is here to serve us. If we want to be the people who can provide these stories for our communities, then we must look after ourselves first. Look at how we operate as individuals (or family units) and how we can maintain our health through a positive relationship with food, water, air, and sunlight.

Through these experiences come the stories that can move the needle in the right direction. People gravitate to solutions that work, and if you can show your community the positive changes you have made to your own life, whether that is through a practice of safe sunlight exposure, production of some fermented sauerkraut, or active breathwork, among other things, they may be interested to learn more and give it a go themselves.

This brings an end to the first part of this book. We have looked at the first four practices: food, water, air and sunlight. The elements. All of them are a prerequisite for all of humanity. As we finish talking about the elements, I want to invite you to take a moment the next time you are outside to stop and pause. Take a breath in for five and out for five. Be thankful for this beautiful world that we are lucky to live in.

We will now look at movement, mindfulness, and sleep, the last three of the Seven Practices.

Seven Practice Recommendations

- Get out in the morning sun
- Use the app dminder to inform safe sunbathing
- Ditch the sunglasses
- Make an outdoor workspace
- Let natural light inside your home
- Spend 15 minutes outside every day
- Find out when natural vitamin D is available in your country

PRACTICE 5
MOVEMENT

EVER SINCE THE first single-cell organisms started to react to sunlight, converting solar energy for their uses, movement became a necessary tool for survival.

Millions of years of evolution have relied on our ancestors, in whichever shape that was, to move through their landscape, hunting and foraging other life forms as they went. All creatures are naturally connected by their desire to use movement to enhance their survivability.

Since birth, we have not stopped moving. Even in the most sedentary moments, the cells within our bodies are constantly moving and interacting as part of their normal behavior.

When sleeping, our bodies still use energy to keep everything functioning, from the blood pumping around the body to the rising and falling of the diaphragm as it controls the breath. And similar to breathing, with movement, we can either sit back and go through our lives with a passive relationship to it, such as only getting up to answer the door, walking to the car or around the local supermarket. Or we can build an active relationship with movement, such as cycling instead of getting the bus or opting for an evening walk rather than a sofa session.

With tools like the internet at our disposal, it is now possible to remain in our homes indefinitely, rarely moving beyond our own four walls.

As we retreat into the digital world, we risk losing what it is to be human. Of course, the ability to connect digitally will play a major factor in our lives in the future, but it cannot consume our society beyond a certain point. To spend more time in the digital world than the physical world is to risk starving our body of the stimulation it may need to survive, let alone thrive.

Responsibility to our Body

In just 11,000 years, our interaction with food and water systems has been domesticated beyond recognition for the ease of human consumption. As populations grew, agriculture gave many people freedom from the daily activity of growing food.

For most of us, the gathering of food and water through physical effort is no longer necessary, and the gathering of its replacement, money, can be earned through activities requiring little to no movement.

We can fight against it by building gyms and promoting yoga, but the reality is that a growing number of humans are simply not moving enough. It is not adequate to move our bodies just enough to survive. We have to move enough to give our bodies the feedback they need to thrive.

As humans, we have a responsibility to our bodies to move regularly. Similar to what we eat, how we move, breathe and drink, directly influences our well-being.

The relationship we have with our bodies must be nurtured. We have an innate connection to our bodies' movement; even with our eyes closed, we can sense our limbs. Proprioception, sometimes considered our sixth sense, is the ability to sense our limbs without sight.

Try this now, put one arm out wide, close your eyes and slowly bring your index finger to the tip of your nose. Even without vision, most of us can sense where our limbs are and touch the tip of our noses. If that is too easy, the next step is to close your eyes and try to touch both index fingers together instead.

We are a marvel of evolutionary biology, and we must not let our domesticated environments dull our senses. The more we move, the better we are at proprioception and the better the link between mind and body.

The great thing about the Seven Practices is that they are intuitive. You and only you know whether you could be moving more or less. If you are honest with yourself, are you working towards the couch potato or the supple leopard?

THE BODY ADAPTS

The human body is a marvel of adaptation and is capable of finding a way to move through a myriad of physical challenges. Through practice and consistency, the body can adapt in many ways.

Footwear

A drastic example of adaptation occurred in China when foot binding was widespread amongst women. Foot binding is where people, primarily young girls, restrict the growth of their feet to increase their perceived attractiveness.

Foot binding is accomplished by bending the four small toes under the foot and wrapping them for up to a month at a time leaving only the big toe pointing forwards.

The result of foot binding is a toe shape unlike that of a normal human. The smallest toes are bent underneath the foot, with just the big toe pointing forwards.

Now what you just read might sound awful, and you may think there is no way you would ever put your feet through it. But I would bet that most people reading this book wear footwear with a similar, albeit less drastic, effect on their feet.

Throughout the modern world, brands like Adidas, Nike and Reebok dominate the movement scene. Since the middle of the 20th century, when Phil Knight released the first running shoe, athletes have been following Nike's every innovation.

As Nike shoes helped runners get faster, other brands started to mimic the design. This has resulted in an industry focused on fast times at any consequence. We are developing shoes that might help athletes to run faster, but at what cost?

In the sportswear industry, among other industries, most shoes restrict the true nature of the foot. I know first-hand the impact this can have on the development of feet as I struggled with bunions at the age of 25. Over 20 years of wearing small shoes that did not respect the true nature of my foot caused the muscles in my feet to atrophy from a lack of engagement. This resulted in the entire bone structure of my foot changing. The widest point of my foot was no longer at my toes; it was at the ball of my foot.

I ask you to take a look at your feet now. Where is the widest point?

I hope the answer is at your toes. But more than likely, you are in the same boat I was, and the widest point is at the ball of your foot. Just this adaptation alone totally goes against millions of years of evolution. In just 50 years, the footwear industry has single-handedly dismantled one of the beautifully evolved aspects of being human; the foot.

If we break down the design faults of modern shoes, it becomes obvious why our society is facing so many issues with our feet, back, knees and hips. The typical trainer includes a heel drop, where the foam sole is padded disproportionately to the back of the foot. By wearing these high-heeled trainers to run in, you are instantly reducing the ability of your calves to cushion the impact.

Your lower leg is designed to work as a big spring with tension going from the tips of toes, up the ankle and then up the calves, where the tension is then used to bounce you back into your next stride. This becomes harder the greater the heel.

Furthermore, when your heel is higher than your toes, it encourages the heel to land first during a stride—again completely negating the ability of the foot, ankle, and calf to absorb the tension.

Think about when you are on tiptoes. You can constantly adjust your height by going up and down on your toes. Compare that to standing on your heels, where there is no option to adjust your height between foot and knee.

By landing on your heel while running, you send the full impact of that stride up the calf and then onwards into the knee, unsurprisingly an area where many runners suffer from injury.

It is not just the high heel of these trainers that causes damage to the foot. The toe box size is also responsible for adapting the shape of the toes. For years I wore size seven shoes without knowing how my feet were supposed to look, and I did not realize the impact I was having on my feet.

Wearing shoes with a small toe box is like wearing boxing gloves on your hands. Imagine putting boxing gloves on every day that crammed all our fingers together and restricted them from moving. Would you be surprised when your hands start failing to work as nature intended?

By shoving our toes into these unnaturally small toe boxes, we are encouraging the big toe to develop pointing inwards, leading to the joint for the big toe protruding outwards—voila, a bunion.

Everywhere we look in our society, you see shoes designed without any consideration for the human foot.

In the fashion industry, people are asked to wear shoes that manipulate their toes into a tiny space whilst requiring their heels to be five inches off the floor. When did that become normal?

Many people wear shoes like this to work every day for most of their lives, sometimes suffering from permanent foot damage as a result. My wife even managed to rip the ligaments in her left foot, twisting her ankle while wearing high heels (before she began wearing barefoot shoes).

Although not quite to the same degree, we practice our own kind of foot binding every time we cram our feet into smaller and smaller shoes. From trainers to high heels and brogues to boots, we are experiencing a global footwear pandemic.

It is no surprise that we are a society of poor movers compared to our ancestors if the two things we move around on are being so distorted from what nature intended.

Destructive shoes may always have a place in our society in elite sport or fashion, but there must be a balance with time given to your feet operating naturally. Wear your fancy trainers to race in, but do not wear them every time you train. Wear high heels to go to a wedding, but do not wear them to work every day.

Since I started rewilding my feet in 2017, I have gone from a UK size seven shoe to a UK size nine shoe as my toes have spread out, and my feet have started to return to their ancestral shape, thanking me for it.

My journey with footwear was personal, and I tell it to inspire others to go on their rewilding journey. You may wish to try some of the suggestions I am going to make, but you may also wish to take your own path entirely.

Firstly, I invested in Correct Toes dividers. These dividers are designed to be worn with or without shoes and look similar to the foam dividers people use whilst painting their toenails. The dividers encourage your toes to operate in their natural position, encouraging the foot's natural movement to take place. I wear them to work, in the gym, to the shops and even on our week-long wild camping trips.

Secondly, I started the long process of replacing my damaging and domesticated footwear with shoes that have a wide toe box and no heel (zero-drop). The shoe brands that I now choose to wear include Vivobarefoot, Vibram Five Fingers and Xero Shoes. I still have shoes from other companies, but only those pairs have a wide enough toe box.

Qualifying as a Vivobarefoot Barefoot Coach helped me to coach my feet, building well-aligned posture and technique to avoid injury. It encouraged me to take my journey slowly, prioritizing barefoot time in nature. It can be easy to avoid this simple step, opting to keep shoes on in nature, whether barefoot or not. But from my perspective, barefoot time in nature is the leading reason that my toes are returning to their natural state. Nothing beats the feedback you get with your feet connected directly to the ground.

After making these changes, my feet have begun to operate more naturally. I have also adapted my walking gait, no longer bypassing my little toe when I walk or run, and you can see that change in the way the soles on my shoes now wear down.

Whenever I buy shoes now, I take the insole out and stand on it. If my toes do not have adequate room when standing on the insole, I do not buy the shoe. It is simple as that.

Another course I recommend for anybody looking to rewild their feet is the Outside Edge by Tim Schieff. This course helped me to reconnect with the outside edge of my feet, as nature intended. In the course, Tim provides a range of movements and instructions to help us get back to our wild walking gait.

The only silver lining I can see from this global experiment with footwear is that the body will adapt. You put it in a bad situation, and it will do its best to learn a new way to get from A to B. However, you put it back in a good situation, and it will do its best to repair too. We are born into a body that has evolved to move, and when we limit our movement, we also limit our potential as humans.

Everyday Movement

Not all of us love throwing weights around a gym, but there will be something out there that you enjoy.

Anything from samba to skiing and dancing to diving will give your body the feedback it needs. Try new things, and step outside your comfort zone. The worst thing that happens is you meet new people you may not have met before and learn a bit more about yourself.

Amber and I hike up and down mountains and through forests with heavy backpacks, which is not for everyone! When you find a movement practice you enjoy, you will be looking after both your physical and mental health.

A bonus is if you find something you enjoy that gets you out of breath. Every time you get out of breath you push your physical limits, growing your capacity for physical health. Get out there, get moving!

To capitalize on more marginal movement gains, I challenge you to adapt your workspace to encourage everyday movement. I want to encourage all desk workers to rethink their work environment. If you have the space and means, create different workspaces that allow you to sit and stand differently throughout each day.

I have a desk for delivering online talks and a standing and ground sitting desk for other work. I use all three of these desks daily, going between my ground sitting and standing desks most often.

The trick here is to keep moving. If I spent all day at my standing desk, I would likely be doing the same damage as sitting all day. Have fun and get creative with your workspace. You do not need a fancy stand to make a standing desk. A pile of books will work just as well.

LIFE IS MOVEMENT

Many things in life operate best when they are balanced, and movement is no different. While it is not possible to be moving at 100 percent all day every day, it is also not adequate to lead a sedentary lifestyle 24/7.

There is no expectation from me that everybody who reads this book has to go out and run a couch to 5k. I would not even recommend it. But there are some changes we can all make in our day-to-day lives to encourage our bodies to move.

Feedback

Our modern world is designed with convenience at heart, with comfort a close second. As the world connected and the global market grew, each of us gained the freedom to be less worried about Maslow's Hierarchy of Needs hygiene factors, such as shelter and safety.

As more people gain simple access to the fundamentals of life (food, security, and shelter), they become capable of concentrating on life's comforts. Around the world, there is now a growing demand for products that can make our lives more comfortable.

On the one hand, we are creating a world where our every luxury has already been considered and will be provided—for a price, of course. And on the other hand, we are facing the extinction of one of our most ancient skill sets: movement.

Activities and movement patterns that came so naturally to all of us as children have been replaced by cars and chairs as we grow older. Our ancestors walked around barefoot, sat on the floor, threw rocks, hung from trees, swam in lakes and carried heavy packs hundreds of miles.

That is our natural playground, and that has been our day-to-day activity for the majority of our evolution. Scientists now believe that the brain itself was only able to develop to its current point because our ancestors needed to move.

It is believed that over time, as the need for complex movements increased, natural selection favored those of us with larger brains, more capable of performing complex tasks that engage many different parts of the body.

As builders and problem solvers, we have always been looking for the next innovation, the next tool that can help humanity.

One tool has become so popular and synonymous with our daily lives that it now outnumbers humans on the planet. Each of us has likely used one of these every single day of our lives, and you will have many of them in your home. You are probably using one right now.

The tool I am talking about is the chair. Used daily by most of our society, the chair has become one of man's most popular inventions.

When I say chair, I do not just mean the seat with the back. I refer to all forms of the seat, whether a bench, stool or something else. We have created a wide range of products that allow us to sit for long periods without feeling the urge to move—something our ancestor's bodies never had the luxury of. Our bodies adapt to any situation we put them in, and now that we can be sedentary for longer periods than at any other point in our history, our bodies are getting good at it.

The use it or lose it saying applies directly to this situation. Human bodies across the globe are losing the ability to perform many basic movements, from walking and running to flat foot squatting and hanging.

Everything in the human body works on a feedback system, A lack of stimulation causes human tissue to break down over time—think bed sores. Chronic inactivity leads to a degeneration of physical capability across the entire spectrum and a marked increase in physical and mental health risks.

Research into physical activity from Professor Steven Blair at the University of South Carolina concluded that physical inactivity is one of the most pressing health problems of the 21st century. Professor Blair recommends that people increase their physical activity to reduce the risk of chronic diseases such as heart disease, type 2 diabetes, and some cancers.[83]

Building a movement practice into your life will positively impact your health over a long-term basis, but it does not mean you have to spend every evening slaving away on the track or in a gym.

A more straightforward way to improve your relationship with movement is to look at the times when you are not moving. Many of us are only active for brief periods, such as travelling to and from work. Even during that travel, some of us will be sitting in a car, train, or another type of transport.

One way to embrace movement during the day is to swap sitting time for standing time. Instead of going straight for the chair on the train or bus, opt to stand up (if you can do it safely), letting your body experience movement through balance. Just like surfing, standing on the train will wake up your ankles, knees, and hips, reminding your body that you are a mover. Or walk up the escalator instead of letting it take you to the top.

For the adventurous, try having a meal sitting on the floor instead of on a chair. It can be eye-opening to experience how challenging it has become to spend time sitting either on our

---

83   Blair SN, 2009

knees or with our legs crossed. For some of us, it may not even be possible right away to assume the cross-legged seated position.

The point is to find the blend between comfort and health. It is no use simply replacing sitting in chairs with sitting on the floor or standing, as all static positions can become detrimental past a certain point. The trick is to keep regularly switching between sitting and standing, encouraging the body to move. The best position is your next position.

The COVID pandemic may have gotten rid of the commute for many people, but it has also freed people to spend that commute time looking after their well-being. If you have swapped your commute for home working, try and get outside in the morning, lunchtime or evening to ensure your body gets the movement it needs.

Natural Movers

When not surrounded by comfort, our bodies fidget as a way of encouraging movement. As we domesticated our sitting habits, our increased comfort helps us bypass the urge to fidget, which results in the atrophy of specific muscles whilst they go unused.

Compare that to using a standing desk where it is easy to instinctively balance from foot to foot and take strolls away from the desk. Just those activities remind the body that it is a mover and that muscles are needed for that purpose.

A life full of micro-movements and adjustments will also support weight loss. People who fidget burn more calories and are typically slimmer than those who spend more time in a state of comfort sedentary.

A study in 2000 showed that when you overfeed people, their bodies start to fight back by increasing fidgeting and posture changes.

Of course, everybody is different, so most people still put on weight in varying amounts. However, the amount somebody fidgeted, strongly predicted how much weight someone might gain. The study showed clearly that the more you fidget, the more weight you lose and keep off. It is estimated that fidgeting can account for up to 1,000 calories of additional burn each day.[84]

In another study, 12,000 women had their fidget patterns analyzed over 12 years. They found that the women who fidgeted more were associated with a lower mortality rate.[85]

Not only has fidgeting been found to improve our overall physical health, but it is also now believed to act as a coping mechanism for improving our mental health. When a group of men were asked to perform a series of mental arithmetic tests in front of an audience, it was the fidgeters among the group that reported feeling less anxious during the quiz.[86]

We do not need to look at our ancient ancestors to see what a good relationship with movement for stress relief was like. There is a plethora of evidence available today, right under our noses.

The wild animals that inhabit Earth use a form of fidget, sometimes described as a tremor, to protect them from long-lasting physiological or psychological damage.

Think about the last nature documentary you watched on the African savannah. Each time the gazelle makes it away from

---

84 Levine, Eberhardt and Jensen, 1999
85 Hagger-Johnson et al., 2016
86 Mohiyeddini and Semple, 2012

whichever big cat fancied it as a meal, they can be seen to shiver along their spine and over their hackles instinctively. This shiver or tremor immediately releases the pent-up stress created by the chase.

Comparing that to humans, we see a similar reaction in people's behavior when smoking. For the smokers or ex-smokers reading this, think of the long shiver you get when you take that first drag. That reaction is no different to the behavior of the gazelle, except they do it instinctively, and we require tobacco cigarettes (or breathwork, as discussed earlier).

Neurobiologist Robert Sapolsky makes the point in his book, Why Zebras Don't Get Ulcers, that zebras, among other animals, are capable of dissipating stress by shaking it off and going straight back to living in the moment.

Compare that situation to modern humans, where the average person carries their emotional baggage with them and sometimes never finds the opportunity to shake it off.

Sapolsky believes that as we develop into adults, we lose this ability to re-calibrate our nervous systems. He says that due to our society's stance that showing feelings are a weakness, we become capable of repressing our genuine emotions, storing them as emotional trauma in our skeletal muscles.[87]

Can you think of a time when you may have done this?

All in all, our bodies have an inbuilt urge to move, and by suffocating all physical feedback, we are making it impossible for our bodies to be well.

We have to pursue discomfort at points in our everyday lives, just as an experiment to see how our bodies react. We are not

---

87 Sapolsky, 2004

at a point in our evolution where we can turn our backs on the physical body that got us here.

We must make conscious decisions about the time we spend in comfortable sedentary and understand that every second on the sofa is a second that our bodies are being neglected.

We are born natural movers. Our bodies develop over nine months of pregnancy with the expectation that we will be born into a world that desires us to move.

I would argue that our toddlers are the best movers in our society. Toddlers only operate at two speeds—run and walk. Like the dog, there is no jogging in the toddler's world. Unlike many adults, they are also capable of the natural rest position of a deep flat foot squat, requiring good ankle, knee and hip mobility and a strong core.

They are also natural climbers and hangers, again requiring the use of their core, whilst hanging gives their entire body a long gravity stretch helping to improve grip strength and joint mobility. These are the activities that the body naturally desires.

We have a responsibility to our children to enable their natural movement as much as possible during their childhood. In many urban areas, roads are dominated by speeding cars, and children are losing their places to play.

For these children, there used to be an element of freedom. They would be allowed to roam the local area meeting new friends and making mistakes on their terms—a critical part of development as a human. But nowadays, many play areas are restricted to organized sports or a mess of metal bars over a domesticated rubber surface.

Freedom of movement for young children has been dramatically restricted as many people no longer have relationships within their communities. One hundred years ago, you may have known all of your neighbors and their kids, whereas many now struggle to have a relationship with even those people living next door.

I do not blame parents for keeping kids inside when the media continues to throw dangerous story after dangerous story into our face about the risks for kids out on the street. But this becomes much harder when there is also no support network of like-minded adults in the community.

However, there is no excuse for the approach to movement at school. Originally a revelation for global organization, the schooling system is now struggling to evolve beyond the reality of children sitting behind lines of desks in either classrooms or auditoriums.

Brian Gaten, superintendent of schools in Emerson, New Jersey, says, "We need to recognize that children are movement-based," and that, "In schools, we sometimes are pushing against human nature in asking them to sit still and be quiet all the time."

Brian and his team have established that it is a fallacy to believe kids are working when they are silent with their heads down. The reality is that children who do not participate in any active time are unlikely to properly energize their brains, making it hard to be productive during those moments of stillness.

The Institute of Medicine filed a report in 2013 showing that regular physical activity can improve a child's mental and cognitive health. The report says, "Children who are more active show greater attention, have faster cognitive processing speed, and perform better on standardized academic tests than children who are less active."[88]

The results of this study will come as no surprise for the theorists who believe the brain developed due to our need to move for survival.

Researchers at Lund University in Sweden corroborated this report and showed that boys who partake in physical activity daily are better performers across the entire schooling curriculum. Movement is now clearly linked to a myriad of educational markers and the development of overall physical health.[89]

In the UK and worldwide, there are schools out there that have taken movement even further. Since the 1990s, parents in the UK have been able to withdraw their children from the traditional schooling system and enter them into forest schooling instead.

The popularity of forest schooling has picked up speed since 2015 as parents have become disillusioned with the outdated methods used in traditional schools.

Regular standardized testing and long periods of sitting, which are commonplace in schools, are counter-productive to raising happy humans. Forest schooling is now seen as an option to encourage children to have a more natural upbringing.

Not designed to run five days a week throughout the year, most forest schools are open typically once a week. The children direct the learning, so the scope of activities is typically broad and varied. Anything from foraging to building shelters, cooking on a campfire, climbing trees, and jumping in muddy puddles can be on the agenda.

---

88 Educating the Student Body, 2013
89 Fritz, 2017

Children who attend forest school have a chance at better physical and mental health as they gain confidence through independence. They have exposure to managing risk, which is essential for learning to trust your body. But importantly, they can build empathy for nature, learning about the sense of place around them and the intricacies of the ecosystem they are a part of. Forest schools encourage children not just to move but to move in nature.

We may have lost wisdom of place from the indigenous people that inhabited the land way before the cities came along, but we have not yet lost the inherent ability of human movement.

If we take the time to see it, there is still a chance for us to learn from all the young humans running around. The next time you tell a child to sit still, consider that they are trying to teach you a lesson: get up and move around. Because that is the human thing to do.

TIME IN NATURE

The body is not very fussy when it comes to movement. However, I find the combination of movement with time in nature the perfect remedy to the busy lifestyle that most of us lead. I wonder what it may have been like 35,000 years ago, to live with all the comforts of our society removed. Our Earth can be a harsh and unforgiving place to make a home, even with all the conveniences provided to us.

Grounding

We have lived in direct skin contact with the Earth for most of our evolution. We may have created footwear, among other tools, that detached us from the Earth occasionally, but much of our lives were spent connecting with the Earth.

We live in the harshest environment faced by humans, but even if we could click our fingers and resolve all of those troubles, the way humans interact with nature still needs to change. We need to do more than heal the planet. We also have to reconnect to nature as individuals.

Throughout humanity's evolution, the Earth's surface has held a negative electrical charge maintained by the thousands of lightning bolts that bombard the planet daily. When the human body is in direct contact with the Earth, it can gain the same electrical potential, improving the health of various bodily processes with it. This is called grounding.

However, most modern buildings insulate us from the electrical energy outside and expose us to various man-made electrical charges indoors instead. This leads to our body experiencing an absence of electrical energy from the Earth.

New research, which has grown substantially since the beginning of the 21st century, is looking at the benefits of having a natural skin-to-Earth relationship. It is now believed that when we spend time with a direct skin connection to the Earth, we can gain positive effects from the electrical charges that the Earth generates.

In a small ten-person study, scientists looked at the benefits of exposing yourself to direct physical contact with the Earth over a 2-hour period. Subjects were grounded using conductive patches attached to their hands and feet. These patches were then attached to a small stainless-steel rod inserted into the Earth outside. They were then asked to sit in a comfortable reclining chair in a sound-proof room for 2 hours.

Measures of their red blood cells taken after the experiment showed a clear increase in their surface charge compared to samples of red blood cells from before the experiment. This increase in the surface charge of our red blood cells, through grounding, makes our blood become less viscous or clumpy, significantly reducing the risk of cardiovascular disease.[90]

Maybe one of the reasons why there is such a passionate love for the beach is because when we are there, we spend more time earthed to the sand and the sea. This has the potential to improve our mood and overall health, making us feel better (vitamin D from the sun will play a part too).

Over time, maybe we as a human race begin to associate the beach with nicer and nicer thoughts, and after generations, we no longer know why we like the beach just that we do. It is likely that even though we have only just learnt the science, our bodies have guided us towards what is healthy for a long time.

The science is great to know. I like to understand objectively what is happening, if possible. If only to help me find the most effective solution to rewilding parts of my domesticated life. The invention of science would have had massive ramifications for the behavior of early humans, who had not yet built a name for themselves as the pattern predictors they would go on to be.

Nowadays, each one of us is looking for patterns everywhere. Subconsciously or not, we are trying to explain away every little thing that happens, putting it down to something or other, just to add a little bit of order to our world.

90 Chevalier, Sinatra, Oschman and Delany, 2013

Sensory Overload

Imagine being a hunter within a community 40,000 years ago with the collective responsibility to feed between 30 and 150 people. To forage water daily, you walk down to the river, collecting berries, roots, and firewood along the way. While walking to the river, you inspect the game trails to see what animal life is neighboring your camp.

Your tribe's survival is based on the berries and roots collected from the river drainage, but for the tribe to thrive, you need to access to protein from the animals on the land.

Each day you examine the game trails, you learn a little more about what they are telling you, and then one day, when you are out hunting with the group, you spot a blood marking on a tree that is very similar to something you have seen before. The last time you saw that sign, there was a boar in the area that had been hurt.

You explain this to your fellow hunters and say that you believe a hurt boar is just behind a tree a short distance downhill. At first perplexed, your fellow hunters choose to listen to you as you are the most experienced hunter in the group. Miraculously to the group, you were right, and the boar is harmed and lying exactly where you predicted.

Just like that, humans started to use the first science, the science of tracking. This skill continued developing instinctively as our ancestors improved their tracking methods, allowing them to find deeper meaning and understanding of the area where they built their homes. The success of our ancestor's hunting skills within these wild places is why we are all here today.

This is the experience I look for from my time in nature. No, not tracking an injured boar, but a complete sensory overload, so deeply felt that it is hard to focus on anything other than the current task.

I am not worrying about my mortgage when looking for the ripest damson berries to pick for my next gin. And I am not worried about next week's job interview when I am crossing a river. Nature is one of life's most engaging distractions and can be a great tool to distract busy minds.

Being out in nature and spending time with ancestral movements like the flat foot squat and walking barefoot will help us continue to rewild our domesticated movement patterns.

To regain confidence in our bodies' physicality will require us to keep seeking discomfort and putting our bodies into situations where they can receive movement feedback. Only through stressing the body will it be possible to rediscover our physical potential.

We will start to heal when we treat sedentary moments with care, frequently repositioning and fidgeting. If we can find the right blend, we will be ready to reap the benefits of a sedentary society without disabling our innate movement ability.

Use restorative rest positions like the flat foot squat and the cross-legged sit to support the body's recovery and aid our ability to grow as movers.

I challenge anybody currently incapable of a flat foot squat to keep practicing. It took me about two years of practice before I could effectively flat foot squat again, just like when I was a child. To get started, I used the edge of a rug under my heels, making it easier to get into that deep squat position. But anything that raises your heels slightly will work.

We do not need to spend every second of every day in an awkward yoga move or eat every meal sitting on the floor.

As long as we actively manage our relationship with movement, humanity's future as a species of movers will be safe. In a time when we do not yet completely understand the impact that a sedentary life will have on the future of humanity, we must find a way to reconnect with our ancient ancestors and aim for individual achievement of our movement potential.

Seven Practice Recommendations

- Look at the toe boxes and heels of your shoes
- Ground barefoot in nature
- Find an enjoyable movement practice
- Swap sitting time for standing time
- Practice the flat foot squat and hanging
- Find a spot to move in nature
- Walk barefoot more

PRACTICE 6

MINDFULNESS

WE HAVE SEEN the importance of movement, and for the sixth practice, mindfulness, we will continue to look at how we can build an awareness of positive well-being.

The body and the mind are synonymously linked, and I cannot see a future for humanity that does not include both an active approach to movement and an active approach to mindfulness.

Mindfulness was introduced to the western world by Thich Nhat Hang, a revered Zen master of Buddhism and Jon Kabat-Zinn, an American professor of medicine. Kabat-Zinn created the Mindfulness Based Stress Reduction (MBSR) program that many people regard as one of the foundations of western mindfulness.

Positive, Present, Proactive

I like to talk about mindfulness as any moment you find yourself able to step away from your constant stream of thoughts and either consider where they are coming from or be aware of no thought at all.

For me, mindfulness can happen in the gym, on the train, lying in bed, and almost anywhere else. Mindfulness as a well-being practice is about being present, positive, and proactive. These are the three words I want to guide you on your mindfulness journey.

For as long as documented history, people have used mindfulness to calm the mind. But, for many humans alive today, it is one of the most neglected of the Seven Practices.

DISTRACTED WORLD

Choices, choices, choices. In this digital age, we have become accustomed to having many options at our fingertips.

I mentioned the book Sapiens earlier, and in his second best-selling book Homo Deus, Yuval Noah Harari compares the human being's thought process to that of an algorithm, simply exporting decisions based on data that has been input. He paints a picture of a world where the pattern of each human's experiences can explain their every decision.

He believes that computers will get to the point where they can document our unique experiences in such detail that they may well be capable of making our decisions. A scary prospect.

Technology

Technology certainly has the potential to continue revolutionizing how each one of us live our life. But until the iPhone can make every decision for me; my brain will still have to pull its weight.

Our "switched on" society allows no reprieve from the endless bombardment of information. Smartphones and watches make distraction a constant feature of daily life as our senses are bombarded by flashing lights and electronic sounds.

Technology has moved along step-by-step. It only makes sense that once we had invented the technology to communicate from afar, it would proliferate worldwide. For a species of animal that has evolved to communicate in groups, the invention of a technology that allows us to communicate with whomever we want has been nothing short of a miracle.

No longer restricted to face-to-face progress, the global connectivity switch on has allowed humans to network globally, pooling together information to increase the speed of innovation to the current rate.

However, our current innovation only seems to be aimed at increasing the time we use our devices for, with not much to do with the quality of that time.

In 2020, over a third of people around the entire globe owned a smartphone. Over 3.5 billion people around the globe now own a phone, and around 1.5 billion new phones enter the market each year. If you include all the smart devices we use, there are currently over 10 billion in circulation—more than the entire population of humans.

Like how chairs managed to take over the world, drastically outnumbering humans, smart devices appear to be growing in dominance too.

These results may encourage companies like Apple, Amazon and Google to continue building a new normal around the connectivity of smart devices. But I am conflicted about the rate of progress we are experiencing right now. On the one hand, I feel so proud to be a member of a society capable of performing the technological feats we now see each year. But on the other hand, I am concerned that the rate of change may be too fast and that we risk severing our connection to the physical world even more.

As humans, we must ensure that we honor the evolutionary steps it has taken to reach this point, regardless of the technological innovation we are capable of. We are on the cusp of losing our concentration to these devices, and we must consider what we might lose if that happens.

It has long been known that repeated interruptions can damage our ability to concentrate. And one of the most documented disadvantages of being constantly connected is increased levels of distraction.

In 2005, research at London's Institute of Psychiatry found that persistent interruptions at work or home can significantly affect productivity.[91] Just two years later, the first iPhone was released, and since then, smartphone users from around the world have been part of an unofficial global experiment to see if humanity can maintain its concentration in a switched-on world.

We no longer have just phone calls and emails to worry about. We also have interruptions from our favorite social media accounts, football teams, clothing brands, video games and many more.

Companies no longer require traditional external marketing to advertise as their apps allow them to post content directly into our personal news feed. Nowadays, our news feeds can be bombarded by countless notifications vying for our attention before we have even woken up.

Historically, our "news feed" may have been something as simple as a mailbox or a pigeonhole at work. But nowadays, our feed can disseminate information from all across our lives.

---

91 Wainwright, 2005

Companies can even use this space, if you let them, to compete against your friends and family for your attention.

In 2002, it was estimated that the average person is distracted in work up to 60 times. And that each of these distractions take you away from your primary job for an average of 5 minutes. This means a massive 5 hours spent in work were spent in a state of distraction.[92]

Just think how much worse it has gotten since then. The average person's smartphone sends about 45 push notifications a day, each capable of damaging concentration. Not only that, but according to Ofcom, people in the UK check their phone every 12 minutes regardless of whether it has pinged or not.

The concerning pattern we see is that the more we let our phones dictate our focus, the better they get at doing it.

Linda Stone, an ex-employee of both Apple and Microsoft, coined the term continuous partial awareness (CPA) to describe the current state many smartphone users find themselves in.

Stone says that in the short term, humans can be remarkably capable of adapting to the always-on lifestyle of many smartphone users. However, over time, the body has to produce increased levels of adrenaline and cortisol to maintain that always-on and alert state, which can begin to cause physiological harm.[93]

Our body can respond in the same way to a smartphone notification as the body of our ancient ancestors would have when faced with predators or threats in their environment. Our society may now protect us from the physical risks that many humans faced during our evolution, but it is not protecting

---

92 Griffey, 2018

93 Stone, 2022

us psychologically from the risk of constant technological connection.

I want to paint a picture of a world where the heart does not drop mid-task because you spot your boss' name on an email notification. A world where your attention is more important than to be drawn away each time a friend double taps your new Instagram upload.

I want us to all build a relationship with technology that puts us in control, not the other way around.

Right now, our bodies are adapting to a life of distraction. However, there is still time to stem the flow and move the needle back towards a life of concentration by adapting our relationship with smartphones and technology.

All it took for me to take back some control was to turn off push notifications for most applications.

Right now, the only notifications I receive are phone calls and messages. It has been great to have a relationship with notifications where each time my phone vibrates, it is because a human person, whom I more than likely know, has sent me a message. No more Instagram, Twitter or Mail notifications mean that I now choose when to use each of those apps, rather than them choosing when they want my attention.

It is not just the distractions we choose that find their way into our thoughts. Outside of our smartphones, we are still bombarded by advertising everywhere we look.

I remember going to Niagara Falls in Toronto, Canada and on the American side of the falls, each building was topped with large advertising boards. Even in Niagara Falls, advertisers on the American side are fighting for our attention.

Clearly, this form of advertising is successful. Otherwise, we would not be living in a world full of billboards. However, some communities around the globe are now wising up to the impact that advertising is having.

In 2006, the mayor of Sau Paulo, Brazil, took drastic action and passed the "Clean City Law." This law prevented advertising on billboards, trains and in front of shops.

Critics believed that removing advertising in the city would result in the loss of over 20,000 jobs and $133 million in revenue. However, this did not prevent the law from passing, and 15,000 billboards were removed from the city upon enactment.

After five years of the ban, over 70 percent of residents reported finding the ban beneficial, with the removal of advertising space reconnecting the Sau Paulo citizens to the historical architecture of their city.[94]

Similar initiatives can be seen in other parts of the world. In Bristol, England, a group called Adblock Bristol worked with their community to oppose billboards and other corporate advertising, suggesting that their city should reflect local culture, supporting the unique identity of its community.

Bristol is a city home to many local shops, and by limiting the number of billboards typically dominated by large corporates, they are working towards a future where more money will circulate in the local area, increasing economic activity throughout the city.

---

94 Curtis, 2011

Multitasking

A healthier relationship with advertising is a great way to get back some of the focus we have lost in this distracted world. But it is not the only thing we can consider if we are looking for a life of concentration.

One of the biggest myths about concentration is the impact of multitasking on productivity. Simply, there is no such thing as multitasking. Instead of multitasking, what we are actually doing is rapidly changing our focus between two different tasks.

It has been scientifically proven that our attention can only be in one place at any time, so it really is one task or the other. Of course, switching tasks is fine, and we will often have to alternate between different jobs. However, to improve concentration in the moment and in the long term, we must manage how often our attention moves between tasks.

Just like limiting the number of push notifications vying for our attention, we also have to consider how many times we jump between different tasks.

Changing how we work can be seen as a drastic step for some, with many professionals having built up their ways of working over long careers. However, the hidden side effects of multitasking are real, and by going back to focus on one task at a time, we can begin to reconnect with the levels of concentration that we were capable of only a generation ago.

Simply put, if you need to think about something, do not do anything else at the same time; give that task your entire focus. Remember, we are not productivity machines. Where you can, take breaks away from the screen. Go outside. Reset your creativity in nature. Each mindful break from work will help the brain analyze and refocus on the task when you get back to it.[95]

Our society has two paths ahead of it: one is a world of concentration where humans can actively and creatively engage with any task they choose, and the other is a world of distraction where humans never reconnect with their creativity; choosing to consume the world given to them rather than create the world they want.

This choice starts with each one of us in each moment. Every time that smartphone pings, do you want it to be a loved one reaching out or an online shop trying to sell you their new summer range?

We humans have value, and we must realize that advertisers worldwide are fighting for our attention. When we are presented with phone notifications we did not choose, consider whether that app is what we want, taking up space in our news feed. If not, turn off the notifications.

Marketers and advertisers worldwide are relying on you to lose concentration so they can grab your attention. If we respect our attention and where we place our concentration, we will find a way to navigate through this distracted world.

Do not just delete those annoying emails. Unsubscribe and save yourself the distraction next time.

ACTIVE OR PASSIVE

Finding a way through the distractions of modern life is tough. A healthy relationship with technology and a focused approach

---

95 Mark, Gonzalez and Harris, 2005

to productivity can go a long way. But we must also find ways to connect with what we truly enjoy.

To do this, we must consider how we live our lives. We can all make the effort to be more present in our lives. Being present means managing our focus and minimizing the impact of distractions. When we are focused, we are actively approaching our lives. However, when we are impacted by endless distractions, bouncing from task to task, we become more passive, allowing outside influences to impact our attention.

How present are you?

Do you approach your life actively, trying to be in each moment?

Or passively, watching time run away from you?

Mindset

In Mindfulness, our mind is sometimes referred to as the "wandering mind" simply because that's what minds do. When this happens whilst trying to be mindful, we can gently bring the mind back by focusing on breathing or refocusing on the present.

Noticing that the mind has wandered off is in itself mindful and is often the first stage of becoming more mindful.

We can all build the presence of mind to step back from our thoughts, assess where they may be coming from, and consider why they may have been triggered.

Connecting to our thoughts is a step toward being present and understanding how to support our well-being. When we slow down and approach our life actively, we allow our mind to perform as evolution intended.

One study at North Carolina State University asked people to participate in a 15-week online program that used planned behaviors to help alter their eating habits.

The participants were divided into two groups, one group behaved as usual, but one group was asked to start planning mealtimes and snack breaks. During those meal sessions, they were asked to concentrate on the food they were eating, consider the taste of each mouthful, and reconnect with the experience of eating.

Upon conclusion of the study, the members of the mindful eating group had lost on average, 5 pounds, compared to an average loss of 0.5 pounds in the control group.[96]

Our brain is not as clever as we want it to be. We think we can quickly eat a salad whilst sitting in rush hour traffic on the way to our next meeting, and there will be no consequences.

This is not the case. We have stopped putting a price on the value of experience. I always thought that if the right food went in my mouth, my body would physically fall into place. But it is not as simple as that. We must also slow down and think about the entire experience to get the most from our food.

Professor Hermann Toplak, President of the European Society of Obesity, asks people to de-stress before mealtimes. Professor Toplak says: "Reducing stress before eating is one of the most important things. If you have stress in your job, don't go [straight] home for dinner."

When was the last time you considered your stress levels before a meal?

---

96 Knowles, 2018

Professor Toplak says that food choices directly reflect stress levels and that in cities like London, where people are more stressed on average, the eating experience is typically quicker and sweeter—and not the good kind.

When you eat purposefully, you are eating without distraction; when you are without distraction, you practice mindfulness.

Mindful eating means paying attention to each mouthful and how the knife and fork feel in your hand as you use them. It means turning off the TV or the computer and putting down the phone to concentrate on how fortunate you are to have a meal in front of you.

The religious practice of saying grace can be a mindful way to ground your thoughts before a meal. By being thankful for all the ingredients and people that came together to create the meal in front of you, you are putting your mindset into a place of positivity where it is most capable of gaining health and well-being from the food.

A common way to practice mindfulness and active eating is a raisin meditation. A simple meditation that aims to reconnect people with the practice of active eating, the raisin meditation can be undertaken by anyone at any point (assuming you have some food). If you cannot immediately undertake the meditation, you may want to note this task so that you can return to it later.

The meditation begins by holding a raisin (or any food) in either the flat of your hand or between your index finger and thumb. When holding the raisin, take the time to look at it, focus on its shape and patterns, and notice any imperfections.

The point here is to treat the raisin as if it is the first raisin you have ever seen as you examine its unique features. Begin to feel the raisin, exploring how its texture feels between your fingers or resting in the palm of your hand. Then bring the raisin up to your nose and breathe in deeply, noticing how it smells and how that smell influences what happens in your mouth and stomach. Try closing your eyes during this to intensify the ability of your other senses.

Finally, place the raisin in your mouth and notice how it feels without chewing. Before tasting, take a moment to reflect on what it feels like to hold food in your mouth without chewing—something we rarely do anymore.

When ready, consciously take two bites of the raisin and hold it in your mouth before swallowing. When ready to swallow, try and intercept the automatic reflex and consciously take control of the process, slowly swallowing the raisin. Feel the raisin travel down your throat into your stomach and sense how your body reacts to this small change.

The above is an exercise in focus and attention. This idea is not specific to eating and can be replicated for any manner of tasks, the key being the careful and considered engagement of each sense.

For example, if you were repotting a plant, you would take the time to feel the soil in your hands and smell the flowers as you hold them to your nose. How does the soil feel? How do your fingers know what to do? What does it feel like to move the plant from one pot to another? Where are you sitting? How does that feel?

What about when driving your car? How does the steering wheel feel in your hand? How does the car feel as the wheels rotate to carry you down the road? Are there little bumps on the road's surface, or is it smooth? What else can you hear? Is there wind in the trees or bird songs in the air?

The key is to engage with the present, leaving the past in the past and the future in the future. Finding the presence of mind to engage in your current activity entirely is a simple and easy way to practice mindfulness. When practiced regularly throughout your life, you start training your body to live in the moment and find focus in a distracted world.

The job of refocusing on the present is not an easy one. One hundred years ago, we simply did not have the technology required for people to be constantly distracted. Without the excess external stimuli, we are surrounded by these days, people would have spent more time alone with their minds. Nowadays, we have a million things to do with our time other than sitting still in our thoughts.

In my lifetime, I have trained my body to expect the dopamine spike that using a smartphone provides. In doing so, I have neglected my thoughts, choosing a life of consuming on a device over time with myself. Just try the next time you are waiting for something to leave your phone in your pocket and just wait. For many readers, it might be surprising how tough this can be. But this is a solid first step to connecting with yourself at a deeper level.

I am optimistic about our future relationship with technology, as I believe that we recognize the impact of being switched on. We must now continue to walk the path that ensures creativity and focus are supported by technology and not the other way around.

Everyday Productivity

Our current idea of being constantly connected and in a mode of concentration is counterintuitive to productivity. By looking at scientists and scholars from the last few hundred years, it is possible to see how drastically different their day-to-day schedules were, despite the scientific acclaim they achieved in their life.

Charles Darwin only worked up to 4 hours a day, despite publishing 19 books throughout his career. Taking the time to begin each day with a morning walk, Darwin would then work in his study between 8:00–9:30 am. Afterwards, he would take a break to read either the latest scientific literature or novel and write letters to his friends and colleagues.

At 10:30 am, he would go back to work for 90 minutes, usually pronouncing his workday over at 12 pm. Darwin would complete his day with an afternoon walk around his home, located just outside London, before returning home for an afternoon nap.

Darwin occasionally returned to his study for another 90 minutes of work between 4 pm and 5:30 pm if he desired. But more frequently, that time would be used for letter writing and leisure.

Darwin's evenings were rarely used for work, and most were set aside for family time. Compare that to the always-on mindset so prevalent among people worldwide. Darwin is not alone, with his fellow prodigies of the 19th and 20th centuries also adopting a more balanced approach to their professional work.

Charles Dickens' son says his father only wrote his novels between 9 am and 2 pm, including an hour for lunch in the middle. After just five hours, Dickens was done for the day.

German author and Nobel laureate Thomas Mann shut himself off daily between 9 am and 12 pm writing his novels, only using the afternoons for reading, napping and some light editing.

Famous British mathematician G.H. Hardy wrote, "Four hours creative work a day is about the limit for a mathematician."

Hardy himself only worked between 9 am and 1 pm, filling his afternoons with tennis and long walks.

So how did we get to the Henry Ford 9–5, and what is the impact on our well-being?

Things have gone so far down the rabbit hole in the other direction now that mere attendance is being used as a marker for productivity. All around the world, people are being quantified for their ability to trade time for money.

As globalization has increased the size of organizations around the world, it has become easier for people to be disconnected from the true meaning of their work. With no opportunity to feel real passion, many people are now simply trading their time for money.

By starving people of their free time and only valuing their attendance as numbers on a sheet, the leaders of global organizations have stripped their staff of the opportunity to develop and perform creatively. We risk destroying the environment required for creativity to grow. In doing so, we put at risk one of the unique elements of what it means to be human.

Torn between the rigorous demands of the modern 9–5 and the continuous bombardment of advertising, the domesticated human of the 21st century is fit to burst with information and expectations.

Fortunately, the modern workplace is catching up. Many employers are now understanding the importance of employee well-being for productivity and engagement. Increasing flexibility, providing suitable benefits and supporting individual growth and development.

When stuck on a creative issue, modern leaders may encourage their staff to go for a walk or catch up with colleagues to encourage creativity.

Our physiology has fallen behind our rate of technological advance. We need to empower society to prioritize mental well-being before we lose our concentration.

We can avoid becoming a distracted society by appreciating the brain's need for mindfulness. We can find our focus again by allowing ourselves time away from society's expectations and focusing on the present.

When we reconnect with our feelings in the present moment, we teach our bodies to operate in the here and now. Even if you practice mindfulness just once a day, this is the first step to taking back control from your distracted mind.

Mark Bertolini, the CEO of Aetna International, an American medical insurance company, initiated a mindfulness program for his company after mindfulness helped him deal with chronic pain after a skiing accident.

Since introducing the mindfulness program, more than one-quarter of Aetna's workforce of 50,000 has participated in at least one mindfulness class, and those who have, reported, on average:

- 28 percent reduction in their stress levels
- 20 percent improvement in sleep quality
- 19 percent reduction in pain

There are also productivity benefits for Aetna, with each employee gaining an average of 62 minutes per week of productivity, estimated to be worth $3,000 per employee per year. An eleven-to-one return on its original investment.[97]

We need to creatively visualize a future where technology works for us as individuals rather than as a tool for propaganda by the leaders of our global organizations and governments. We must seek a utopia that supports creativity and individualism rather than a George Orwell 1984 dystopia focused on distraction and control.

As we will learn later, visualization can make us less anxious and more productive humans. But how we approach the biggest tasks in our lives will define how productive we are. It is easy to procrastinate on our biggest challenges, but I invite you to find the best way to be productive.

Try not to get sucked into easy, quick tasks like emails or social media, especially in the morning. When we start our day with social media, emails or any other quick gratification task, we tell our brain that today is a lazy day; we can put our feet up because we do not need to concentrate.

With many of us instinctively reaching for our phones each morning, think about what you open first and how that will impact your day.

I plan my mornings the night before so I can wake up with a clear plan of what to do. Use your calendars or task lists to prioritize what is truly important to you.

In contrast with the time we spend working, we can also support our mindfulness practice by having a hobby that encourages time in the present.

---

97 Gelles, 2016

My Dad is a passionate windsurfer, and I would argue that he experiences a form of mindfulness whenever he touches the water. It is just him, the board and the sail. With nothing else to distract, he must focus on that moment (it is pretty tough to text while surfing over the waves at 30mph). His experience of windsurfing requires complete and utter concentration, helping him train his mind to maintain focus. Something that can be transferred to all other aspects of our lives.

Of course, it does not have to be windsurfing. Most sports encourage you to focus on the present moment. The golfer concentrating on making par, the dancer performing their routine, and the athlete perfecting their pole vault are all examples of people finding the focus to live in the present moment.

Outside of sports, people find their focus cooking in the kitchen, doodling a picture, playing a game of chess, among many others. There is no limit to where you, as an individual, can find your focus. Bring creativity into your life and explore new hobbies to find what works with you.

VISUALIZE, REALIZE

There are many reasons to visualize a future that you desire. Whether your dream future is to get a new job, find a partner, or travel the world. The practice of visualization will be able to support your work towards that goal.

Purposeful Visualization

Primarily, visualization encourages the brain to take action. When you visualize yourself in a position, your mind's next step is to work out how to get there. If you want to be a bestselling author, you best picture yourself on book tours and podcasts being interviewed about your book (yes, I did that for this book).

To look at it a little differently, just imagine one of your goals in life is to own a campervan, but as things stand, you cannot afford it. Despite identifying the desire to buy the car, you cannot picture a situation where your finances will allow you to make the purchase.

What visualization can do is remove the negative and unwanted thoughts and replace them with constructive ones. Rather than regressing into the frustration of your lack of finances, visualize a future where you have been able to purchase the car. This minor tweak in your thinking means you are now asking yourself, "How can I afford this car" rather than telling yourself you cannot afford this car.

For some, the outcome of the "how can I afford this car" question might be to move house, stop going on holidays or some other financial step you would not be willing to make. However, there may also be a creative solution that comes from asking yourself this question. A solution that, given enough time could lead to you one day owning your dream car.

For many people, our dreams are not out of reach—assuming we truly set our sights on it. When we think with the end in mind, we start to not only picture our deepest desires but also work towards reaching them.

The beauty of visualization is the clarity it can provide you. Once you can imagine the future you desire, you may find the extra inner motivation and passion that makes it possible to reach that target. By focusing on positive goals and visualizing what your life may look like, you can encourage a feedback loop of positive thoughts and drive.

Let me take you on a journey through my visualization. I am wandering through the green canopy of a dense forest in springtime. Sunlight breaks through gaps in the foliage to highlight the occasional patch of Earth on the forest floor.

Beside me are my wife and two of our rescue dogs. We have just begun the 3-mile stroll back to our home after having lunch with neighbors. The weather is warm under the sun but quickly gets cold in the shade, so we break regularly to sip warm tea brewed with local herbs.

On the way home, we take a detour to our local lake for a swim in nature, meeting another couple from our community on the way. After swimming, we all walk back to our tiny house, where we drink homemade apple cider until the late evening.

Due to it being a new moon, we all decide to camp outside under the stars, pitching a couple of tents with just their fly sheets so we can sleep directly under the night sky.

Just like a plan, visualization can be a great way to recognize the path you want to walk in your life. My visualization reminds me that I want to spend time in nature. The most vivid part of my visualization is the greens of the leaves and the browns of the trees. I can see the sunlight as it tries to break through the canopy to reach the forest floor beneath. I can sense my wife beside me as we walk with the dogs through the new growth of bluebells and tulips brought about by the changing seasons.

This is all just part of a larger visualization of my life where Amber-Rose and I find a sense of place in a like-minded community that is sustainable within itself. Only by focusing on this future and genuinely considering what it would look like to be there will we be able to prepare for that eventuality.

I think with the end in mind so I have the skills required to thrive when I get there. I cannot see a future where the core of this visualization does not come true. We might swap the forest for a jungle or the lake for a sea, but at the heart of the visualization is the establishment of our future selves within a community that lives as sustainably as possible.

The power to visualize your future can be one of the most rewarding and exciting uses of human creativity. I find night-time to be the point when my brain wanders the most, and I am capable of my most creative visualization.

Letting my brain have the time to consider what my future self may look like has helped me understand my path more than any book or podcast. One tip I recommend, though, is to scribble down any profound thoughts! You do not want to have forgotten them in the morning.

The plan for this book occurred and evolved during that very same process of active visualization. For the book, I picture people using the Seven Practices to rewild their well-being. I picture a group of passionate rewilders connecting digitally and in real life to share their tales. I picture people reconnecting with their feelings again and building an awareness of their well-being.

This might be new to you, but visualization works, and we can practice it in many ways. One of the world's greatest golfers, Jack Nicklaus, used visualization throughout his career to deliver results on the golf course.

Regarding visualization, Jack said: "I never hit a shot, not even in practice, without having a very sharp in-focus picture of it in my head. It's like a color movie. First, I ‹see' where I want it to finish, nice and white and sitting high on the bright green grass. Then the scene quickly changes, and I ‹see› the ball going there: its path, trajectory, and shape, even its behavior on landing. Then there is a sort of fade out, and the next scene shows me making the kind of swing that will turn the previous images into reality."

Nicklaus uses visualization over a short time frame to encourage his body to deliver the desired result on the golf course for each swing.

Visualization can be used in the short and long term to garner the results you desire from the world around you, molding yourself and your environment.

As someone diagnosed with Crohn's disease at a young age, it became almost a part of my brand. Due to my history of regular infusions, I was incapable of seeing a future for myself where the NHS did not support me. At the time, I believed Crohn's was only curable for 'special' people and that I would be burdened by it for my entire life. There was no forest in my future and no wild food. I never had a clear vision for my future because I knew Crohn's would stop me from traveling and living abroad.

This was the story I told myself repeatedly. I did not think it, I knew it! Without being a doctor or nurse, I had managed to visualize a life for myself that was defined by my illness. Not until 2017 did I take the time to consider how well I truly felt and how my symptoms of Crohn's had stopped flaring up.

Looking back, I can see that I let my illness dictate my vision for the future, closing down my pathway to the wild, forested utopia that I now desire. Even as my health improved, I still tarred myself with the brush of Crohn's disease. Despite improving my physical and mental health during the early days of my rewilding journey, I could not stop labelling myself as somebody with an incurable disease.

People make it into remission for different illnesses every day, and I had not given a second thought that one day I too could be free of the burden of a long-term illness.

I am not telling you to ignore your doctors and nurses; they are the experts in their field, and we need to respect their guidance. But we have to be aware of how we feel as well. Everybody, and I mean everybody, can experience an illness in different ways. Sometimes, we can be our own worst enemy by echoing our fears and concerns back at ourselves—focusing on the negative outcome rather than the positive.

Focus on the positives and visualize a future of health, joyfulness, peace and love.

Gratitude

I remember being so excited to start driving. I was finally turning 17 and able to start my driving lessons. The idea of one day having a car and the freedom that inevitably comes with that was extremely exciting.

However, fast forward five years and driving had become a chore. Gone was the childlike excitement that I used to find behind the wheel, and in its place: boredom and a feeling of monotony.

Driving became so commonplace that I no longer appreciated the many benefits it brought to my life. I could no longer picture my life without the ability to drive, so I was unable to be thankful for my ability to and the fact that I could afford a car.

But the reality is, I am still incredibly privileged. Out of everybody in the world, I was fortunate to learn how to drive safely and afford a car. Sometimes we need to pause and feel grateful for how privileged we are.

The next time you are cleaning your home. Instead of feeling frustrated that cleaning is interfering with what you want to be doing, reflect on the fact that you have a place to call home and the luxury of being able to clean it. Regardless of where your home is, it is yours, and you and your experiences shape it in the same way the experience of living there shapes you.

The reality is, for many people reading this book, we live in a society where we have access to cars and homes, which are generally located in safe neighborhoods with access to both work and community.

We are not trying to be perfect and it does not always work to focus on the positive; cleaning may still feel like a chore sometimes. But, more often, it becomes something that can fill me with pride. Cleaning my home can become a way to inject positivity into my day or break up tasks if I am working from home.

In whatever part we play during our lives, each of us is responsible for visualizing a better future for ourselves, our families and our communities. To visualize a world where everyone has access to nutritious food, clean air and water, and a safe, sustainable place to work, live and play among a community of friends and family.

Mindfulness can be found in everything, and kindness or gratitude makes the positive a priority, allowing us to be present and proactive in whatever way our journey takes us.

Seven Practice Recommendations

- Manage notifications on your phone
- Try the raisin meditation
- Take things one at a time
- Spend time with your mindful practice
- Think of a positive future visualisation
- Write down a gratitude
- Avoid emails and social media first thing when you wake up

PRACTICE 7

SLEEP

THROUGHOUT THE EVOLUTION of humans, no other practice has consumed the amount of time that sleep does. The yin to the day's yang, sleep is our body's way of repairing and recovering. Seen as a pleasure by some and a chore by others, there is a wide variation in the different approaches to sleep taken by different individuals within our society.

Some of us choose to develop a healthy respect for sleep, letting our bodies experience regular sleep for a regular duration. Some of us choose to combat sleep, using stimulants like caffeine to fight off the effects of tiredness. Until very recently, it may have been considered a sign of low productivity to let yourself experience sleep to its fullest, with many successful individuals famously working on less sleep than recommended.

Sleep More

We are in the final chapter of the Seven Practices, and I started with food and ended with sleep for a specific reason. Whilst a relationship with all Seven Practices is critical for a happy and healthy life and well-being, food and sleep could be said to have the biggest impact on the length of life.

A poor relationship with sleep stands firmly next to a poor relationship with food as two of the leading markers for a shorter life. For all our longevity research, simply having a healthier diet and sleep practice can make all the difference to the length of our life.

This chapter will examine why sleep is so important and how we can use time in bed to score free well-being and health benefits.

CIRCADIAN RHYTHM

Over the last 11,000 years, as agriculture has become the dominant method of food production, humans have been required to trade ever-increasing amounts of time to earn income to access food. Compared to humans who used to subsist on a foraged, wild-grown diet, our food now requires work from seed to flower to ensure the crop survives. We have become experts at creating more work for ourselves, and that work is now eating into our sleep time.

Since the conception of agriculture, we have been finding all kinds of reasons to ignore the internal circadian rhythm that our bodies yearn for, fighting against it with lighting and stimulants.

The problem is it is hard for us to self-diagnose sleep deprivation. You can just wake up one morning with sleep deprivation. But it is also something you accrue over time, meaning the most sleep-deprived in our society may not even know. They may take their lack of attention and high stress levels for granted and consider that typical behavior.

Being asleep allows our brain to recover and heal, safely storing memories and actions from the day before resetting afresh for the new day. This is vital recovery time that some of us may need more of.

Sleep Pattern

The body has two prime ways that it triggers sleep in an individual. One is through the neurotransmitter adenosine, and the other is through the signals sent by your circadian rhythm (body clock). The difference between the two is simple: adenosine-triggered sleep is due to energy expenditure, and sleep triggered by the circadian rhythm is simply due to your regular sleeping pattern.

An adenosine triggered sleep may explain why you can be tired in the middle of the day, after a bout of intense activity, even though your sleeping pattern is not adjusted to expect the midday nap.

For many of us, our sleep patterns will be customized to fit our work and play schedules. Some people prefer to sleep early and wake early, spending their free time before work, whilst others will get up for work and spend their free time after work in the evenings.

Your preference for when you sleep is called your chronotype, which will change throughout your life. It is influenced by your genetics and experiences. The Sleep Foundation says, " Generally, most children have an early chronotype. In adolescence, chronotype is pushed back, leading to the myth that teenagers are lazy because they find it difficult to wake up for school.

Chronotype then gradually shifts earlier and earlier upon entering adulthood."[98]

Circadian rhythm looks after many other bodily functions outside sleep, such as body temperature, blood pressure and digestion. It is our responsibility to encourage a healthy circadian clock if we are in the pursuit of well-being. By encouraging our body to have regular sleep at regular times, we can support healthy physiology.

No longer can sleep be viewed as a luxury, or as I have also heard plenty of times—something to do when you are dead. It is an essential part of maintaining both physical and mental health. How we navigate the many disruptions will be different for each of us. But there are still some things we can all do to support healthier sleep.

Lighting

Electrical lighting has been one of our society's groundbreaking technological breakthroughs. Although created initially through a culmination of many people's hard work, it was Thomas Edison's bulb design that would unlock the technology for the masses.

By the beginning of the 1900s, bulbs were mass-produced, and buildings were retrofitted for their installation and use. Although the technology is changing as consumers switch to more energy-efficient lightbulbs like LED, the product is still the same—a bright white light.

In just the last 100 years, electrical lighting has become so synonymous with our society that it has even changed how the

---

98 Pacheco & Rehman, 2023

Earth looks from space. Just like the beautiful rivers and streams that can be seen flowing from the tallest mountains down to the sea, we can now also see the brilliance of electrical light illuminated by the cities reaching to the furthest suburbs and beyond, weaving in that same brilliant fashion that the rivers do.

For me, I cannot imagine a time without electrical lighting. It has been a massive part of my life, and I would feel lost if all electrical lighting was suddenly unavailable. But what does unnatural white light mean for our sleep?

For the first time in our evolution, humans have found a way to turn off the darkness, manipulating day and night as they see fit. Where our sleep was once dictated by the sun, now we are a slave to the bulb, choosing to let glass and filament dictate our sleep instead.

We are using electrical lighting to combat our circadian rhythmicity, which in many different forms has evolved over three billion years to reach us now. We saw in the chapter on Sunlight the importance of spending time outside due to sunlight's health benefits and sunlight plays a significant role in circadian rhythm too.

Since we retreated indoors, our circadian rhythm has suffered from a lack of bright light. As we read earlier, light intensity (lux) is much lower from electrical lighting than the sun. Electrical lighting is just not bright enough to complete a thorough daily reset of our circadian rhythm in the same way as a sunny day. Furthermore, we are now surrounded by lights at night time, swapping the darkness for a perpetual glow. We fondly refer to New York as the city that never sleeps, without a concern for the impact that perpetual daytime could have on its residents.

Is our relationship with electrical lighting impacting our ability to sleep, preventing us from benefiting from the restorative effects of a good night's rest?

Unfortunately, it can be difficult to learn about sleep deprivation because of the ethical issues of inviting people into sleep deprivation.[99] But despite the lack of proper scientific studies since Edison's first bulb design hit the market, it could be said that each of us has been running our own circadian rhythm experiments. When we stay inside, avoid the sun, and are exposed to electrical lighting at night, it can be said that we are choosing to prioritize a pattern that fits our schedule rather than what nature intended.

To understand the long-term impacts, researchers have studied people who work in roles that require them to operate overnight. Nursing and building security are examples of jobs that can be completed during the day or night. Because of this, it is possible to look at the health of individuals who have worked mixed shifts over an extended period and compare that to those who consistently worked night-time shifts instead.

Over the last 20 years, we have collected enough anecdotal evidence of female nurses working alternating shift patterns to confirm a link between disrupted body clocks and breast cancer. When you look at all the data, women who have worked a variable shift pattern over their careers have a higher average number of breast cancer cases.

If you work in a job where you are required to work an alternating pattern of day and night shifts, you may have an increased risk of developing cancer. The worst cases are associated with people continuously alternating between day shifts and night

---

99 Stevens and Zhu, 2015

shifts, with individuals who only ever worked night shifts faring a little better, from a health perspective, over time.[100]

This data was corroborated scientifically when researchers subjected mice to simulated shift work, using lighting to alter their typical circadian rhythm. As expected, the mice subjected to simulated shift work were more at risk of developing mammary tumors.[101]

We are now recognizing that by disrupting our circadian rhythm and running a sleep pattern that fights against the natural rhythm of night and day, we are both increasing the risk of developing tumors within the body whilst also adding additional stress to any other tumors that may be already there.

In mice, the rate of growth increase for a tumor was noted to be as much as two to three times higher in the mice that experienced simulated shift work. The tumors that grew at the slowest pace were always found in the mice with the most robust circadian rhythm.

When I look back on all those times in my life when I stayed up all night, whether at university trying to cram for an exam or as a teenager playing video games, I wonder whether the sleep deprivation I accrued was worth it. If I had known back then the impact that cheating on my circadian rhythm could have, would I still have made that choice?

I want to hope that I would have opted for a good night's sleep instead, but we will never know. What we do now know, though, is that if we can find our circadian rhythms again—as our ancestors did for millions of years—we will give our bodies the best

---

100   Davis, Mirick and Stevens, 2001

101   Van Dycke et al., 2015

opportunity to heal and thrive. We are pattern-seeking creatures, and our physiology desires a regular sleep pattern.

A key to how we can interact with light without damaging ourselves is tied to the lives of those that came before our society. When we look back at our ancestors and their evolutionary path to get us to this point, their lives were intertwined with fire.

Electrical lighting can give off the full visual spectrum of light, with devices like TVs and smartphones broadcasting the entire spectrum of color continuously during their use. Compare that to a fire's deep amber glow, dominated by reds, oranges, and yellows.

During the day, blue light is everywhere. It is found not only in the lighting from our electrical devices but also naturally. For most of our evolution, the primary source of blue light has been the sun itself. This surge of blue light in the midday sun can help support our sleep pattern to align with our natural circadian rhythm.

Think of when you go camping. As soon as the sun sets, you have less unnatural blue light, with the warm glow of a fire and the gentle light of the stars and moon to lull you to sleep. Compare that to the countless devices we are surrounded with at home, each capable of replicating the entire spectrum of visible light.

Even the rightful transition from traditional bulbs such as halogen to more energy-efficient alternatives like LED means we are sacrificing sleep-friendly amber lighting for the blue lighting that LED typically gives off.

All this light pollution is telling our bodies to stay awake, that it must surely still be daytime.

Our bodies become even more confused when we do not venture out in the day, as the lack of quality light in the home means our circadian rhythm does not reset in the morning either.

If we stay inside and surround ourselves with technology in the mornings and evenings, it can be impossible to find the ancestral sleep that our bodies deserve and desire.

Companies like Low Blue Lights have been trying to capitalize on this since the early 2000s. Following on from research suggesting that the blue light within the visible spectrum of light can alter our circadian rhythm drastically, they designed a pair of tinted sunglasses to minimize the blue light that reaches our eyes.

Science says that we are suffering from an inability to produce melatonin due to the constant interruption of blue light during what should be our dark hours. Any exposure to blue light at this point in the day instantly stops the melatonin production. Low Blue Lights argue that their glasses allow the body to produce melatonin during dark hours, as the orange lenses filter out the blue rays before reaching the retina.[102]

These wrap-around orange lens glasses have become a popular product in the biohacking space. Leading biohackers like Dave Asprey are rarely seen indoors not wearing their orange glasses, especially in the evenings. Personally, Amber and I wear Swanwick night-time blue-blocking glasses each evening, putting them on as soon as the sun sets until we get into bed in the dark. They have certainly helped reduce soreness in my eyes and support the evening transition into sleep. We also swapped our evening lighting to amber bulbs.

Electrical lighting is currently winning the battle for our attention. With more and more of our society choosing to put the lights on each evening as the Earth slowly spins on its axis away from the sun, it is even harder to find true darkness

---

102   What LBL Does, 2022

anymore. Our addiction to lighting has become so severe that there are now few places humans inhabit where it is still possible to see the glories of the night sky. Many of us are restricted to looking at NASA's Instagram page to see what our galaxy, the Milky Way, looks like.

Even through a screen, the sight of our galaxy still gives me a sense of wonder. And I cannot help but feel a pang of jealousy that just 300 years ago, witnessing the magic of space would have only required you to look up. It is hard to imagine what it may have felt like to live underneath a blanket of stars each night. And what it would have been like to grow up with an intimate relationship of how they move across the sky each night.

Managing our sleep pattern must become one of the most fundamental practices for our sleep. By finding the right blend between the demands of our modern society and the requirements of our ancient physiology, we can allow the mind and body the time it needs to heal and thrive.

We must be selfish with our need for darkness at night, avoiding blue light in the evening to bring about sleep. And we must be selfish with our light in the day, ensuring we expose our eyes to the brightness of the morning and midday sun.

RECOVERY

Choosing to sleep in line with our ancient physiological desires is one of the keys to unlocking a higher state of wellness. However, simply choosing sleep at any point is likely to allow the body and mind time for recovery.

As a society, we are constantly weighing the value of staying up against going to bed. With more and more to distract us, we try to pigeonhole sleep into this frustrating 8-hour gap between bedtime TV and the morning coffee. However, scientists are now able to objectively put a value on sleep time and show how it enhances the quality of your awake time.

Every year almost 40 percent of countries worldwide take part in a mass sleep experiment as a way of adapting our society's needs to the changing pattern of the sun. This sleep experiment is, of course, the changing of the clocks as the seasons change.

Daylight savings time was created to give people more daylight in the evening and save energy costs. However, we are taking a risk every time we ask people to adjust their sleeping patterns. We can now see from looking at accidents and hospital reports exactly what impact losing an hour's sleep is having.

Losing an hour of sleep may not sound like a big deal to some of you, just a minor inconvenience. But when we look at it across entire populations, that adjustment to our sleeping pattern is enough to increase accidents,[103] heart attacks,[104] miscarriages,[105] and suicides.[106]

Just that small knock to our sleep pattern is tipping certain people past their safe limit. The next time you experience the clocks going forward in spring, remember this and give yourself all the restorative sleep you need. It can take up to a week to adapt to your new sleeping pattern, so give your body the time it needs.

---

103   Coren, 1996
104   Janszky and Ljung, 2008
105   Liu et al., 2017
106   Berk et al., 2008

Sleep Phases

At this point, it is worth knowing two of the different sleep states. REM (rapid eye movement) and NREM (non-rapid eye movement). To achieve a successful night's sleep, the body goes through these different sleep states and their phases. There are three phases of NREM and one phase of REM that we go through on a typical night's sleep.

Stage one of NREM usually lasts for several minutes and is the phase where we can be easily woken. Our brain waves start to slow down, and our muscles start to relax.

Stage two of NREM is when the heart rate and breathing continue to slow down, and muscles relax further. Our core body temperature also starts to drop.

Stage three of NREM is when you start to enter a deep sleep, making it harder to wake up. At this point, your breathing and heart rates are at their lowest. Your muscles are completely relaxed, and the brain waves continue to decelerate.

Stage four is when REM sleep takes over from NREM sleep. This is when eye movement and brain activity increase again, and dreams can occur. In REM sleep, our body is immobile even though the brain is active.

We need NREM and REM sleep to recover physically and mentally after each day. REM sleep will occupy about 20–25 percent of sleep time, with NREM taking up the rest.

How we sleep can be a different experience for everybody, and learning what works will require you to listen to your body. But if we interrupt either stage three or four of our sleep phases, either with an alarm clock or some other interruption, our sleep quality is reduced.

Do not discredit the value of letting your body nap,. For the young and elderly, a short nap in the afternoon of fewer than 30 minutes can alleviate some aspects of sleepiness and fatigue. Whilst the research is less clear about younger adults. I imagine that if you are experiencing a sleep deficit and your body prompts you for an afternoon nap, it can only help your cognitive performance.[107]

In the US alone, 50–70 million people suffer from a sleep deficit, which is expected to be contributing heavily to the increase in the number of individuals experiencing mental health.

Some of us have become so engrossed in our busy lives that we go and go until the late hours of the evening, when finally and reluctantly, we collapse into bed. We have become victims of our distractions, with the tools created to communicate and entertain now so popular that they are taking time away from one of the most fundamental practices of humanity.

Even the urban myth of sleeping for 8 hours a night confuses the situation as each of us has individual needs, and these needs change throughout our lifetime.

Just like we cannot all eat the same food, we all require different amounts of sleep.

To learn how much sleep you need, plan in a week or two, maybe during a holiday when you have no morning interruptions and let your body sleep. Preferably you would perform this experiment rising and falling with the sun. However, the point is to sleep without restriction over a longer period than a weekend, allowing your body to heal and reconnect with its needs.

---

107   Hayashi, Motoyoshi and Hori, 2005

Over the first few days, your body will start to find its preferred waking and sleeping time. When you start sleeping to your pattern, you may find it adapting through the seasons. In the UK, I naturally wake up over one hour earlier in June compared to December.

True Rest

When we give our bodies time to recover through sleep, we also give our brains a boost. Everywhere we look, we are becoming increasingly similar, buying the same clothes, watching the same TV shows and eating the same foods. If we want to combat this slide from creation to consumption, we can use sleep as the spark to light a fire of imagination within us. We are responsible for visualizing our futures, and creativity is one of the most important assets to us for opening up new methods of thinking.

History shows us that sleep can encourage profound breakthroughs. Dr James Watson, the scientist behind the discovery of DNA, is rumored to have uncovered this breakthrough after dreaming about two intertwined serpents with heads at opposite ends.

There is a similar story behind the invention of the sewing machine, with inventor Elias Howe also dreaming of his breakthrough.

As reported by Popular Mechanic in 1905: "One night, he dreamed that he was building a sewing machine in a strange country for a savage king. The king had given him 24 hours to complete the machine and make it sew, but try as he would, he could not make the needle work and finally gave up in despair. At sunrise, he was taken out to be executed, and with the mechanical action of the mind in times of great crises, he noted that the spears carried by the warriors were pierced near the head. Suddenly, he realized that here was the solution of the sewing machine needle. He begged for time—and while still begging, awoke. It was four o'clock. Hastily he dressed and went to his workshop—at nine o'clock, the model of the needle with an eye at the point was finished."[108]

Many other innovators throughout history credit their success to sleep and the dream state that comes with it. The fictional Frankenstein monster and the Periodic table are just two more among many other creations that credit sleep with the reason for their discovery.

What if our society's addiction to a lack of sleep means we miss out on the next crucial discovery to unlock the next wave of innovation?

Just like when we turn computers off and on to fix bugs, we can sleep to improve our creativity and well-being.

Research from the last decade has shed light on what actually happens in our brains during sleep, helping to make sense of why we all benefit so much from a good night's rest.

Scientists Jessica D. Payne from the University of Notre Dame and Elizabeth A. Kensinger from Boston College co-authored an article called Current Directions in Psychological Science. What they discovered is that sleep is making our memories more robust by reorganizing and restructuring those memories, almost like a computer storing files away on a hard drive.

---

108   Jacoby, 2018

This new research shows us that sleep is not only crucial for recovery, but it is also crucial for the storage of new learnings and memories.[109]

As more of us move to home working, maybe we can trade some of the time spent on the commute for more time spent in bed, allowing our brain and body to heal and recover each day.

NATURAL SLEEP

We may all be able to improve our sleep practice. But there will also be some people reading this book who have already built a brilliant relationship with sleep and are simply looking for ways to make their sleep even more beneficial.

One thing we can consider is our sleeping environment. Most of us currently sleep in a room so far from the wild environment that we may just be missing out on those hidden benefits that living in line with our ancestral heritage provides.

To change this, we can experiment with rewilding our sleep for improved health, shunning some of the comforts of our modern society and seeking a more natural environment to sleep in.

Moonlight

For longer than we have been evolving, the moon has circled the Earth, distorting our tides through its gravitational pull. Over a 28-day cycle, we are exposed to different lunar phases and varying light levels depending on how much of the moon reflects light from the sun back to Earth.

---

109   Payne and Kensinger, 2010

Most of us, myself included, have lost our relationship with moonlight, rarely appreciating the moon moving across our night sky. But, for humans and animals that live closer to the natural world, the changing moon can drastically impact daily activities.

Grazing animals such as deer and horses will stay up late into the night during a full moon, using the added light to continue their grazing activities. This can significantly reduce the time they spend exposed during the day, and it is safer for them to be out during a full moon instead.

Imagine how that impacted our ancestors. During a new moon (the opposite of a full moon), their prey would be forced to graze within a greatly restricted window, allowing for less time and effort-consuming hunting.

One of the first standardized tests, designed to look at the impact of the lunar phase on our physiology, took place at the University of Basel in Switzerland.

A key point here is that light exposure was kept the same throughout the test, which meant that all results were linked to just the changing lunar phase and not light levels. Results must also be taken with a pinch of salt, as only 33 individuals were used in the testing.

However, Chris Cajochen and his team laid the foundations for further studies by providing a plausible scientific link between sleep quality and the moon's phases. They discovered that participants slept less deeply and for shorter periods during the full moon than at other lunar phases.[110]

Just like the animals staying up later and grazing during a full moon, it would appear that our bodies also expect some late

---

110   Cajochen et al., 2013

evening hiatus from sleep. We are still at the beginning of a journey to understand how this could be impacting us, but it is worth knowing that in terms of a good night's sleep, you are more likely to have one during a new moon than a full moon, regardless of blackout curtains.

I find it exciting to consider the relationship that my ancestors and, to an extent, I have with the changing patterns of the moon. One of my favorite things to do whilst camping is to watch the moon come up on a clear sky the night of a full moon. It is one thing to experience a sunrise, but another altogether to experience a moonrise, as the light of the full moon brings a pseudo daylight to the night-time dark.

To expand our knowledge, scientists have also looked at the impact of temperature on sleep. If you picture a typical hunter-gatherer tribe in your head, it has long been believed that they would sleep in line with the rising and setting of the sun.

While it is still likely that most would have retired to sleep as soon as the sun went down, it is now believed that most would have risen before the sun rose when the night was its coldest.

Instead of waking when the sun rose, anthropologists now think that the cold of the night could have been the major factor for most rising, rather than the morning light from the sun.

As we settle down to sleep in our climate-controlled home, are we losing yet another factor that may have been playing a part in encouraging healthy sleep for revitalized physiology?

Sleeping in Nature

Just like the circadian pattern of the sun, our bodies have an internal thermostat that follows a similar rhythm, reaching peak internal temperature sometime in the late afternoon and minimum temperature in the early morning hours.

In nature this would happen naturally as the infrared heat from the previous day's sun dissipates slowly overnight, causing a large drop in temperature. However, with most of us now living indoors with the ability to shut out the fluctuating outdoor temperatures, we have to rely on the natural cooling ability of our bodies to get us to the point where deeper sleep may occur easier.

It would be naive of me to suggest that we can all just open our windows, especially for those of you living at extreme ends of the Northern and Southern Hemispheres. But should we be trying to rewild our sleep environments if we want to facilitate the highest quality of sleep possible for ourselves and our families?

Is it possible for you, in the hotter months, to sleep with your window open to experience the natural fluctuations in temperature that your body has adapted to?

How long you sleep will be personal, and you will not know until you experiment. My best night's sleep tends to come from camping out in nature, with long, deep, restorative sleep occurring in winter. Remember, any time we sleep outside, we are embracing airbathing benefits at the same time, truly reconnecting to our wild ancestors.

To summarize our journey with sleep, find a regular sleeping pattern and stick to it whenever you can. Avoid those pointless late nights and lay-ins, and give your body the regular sleep it needs to support your well-being. Sleep in connection with the seasons and camp in nature when possible.

Enjoy the challenge to sleep more and embrace your body's desire to rest and recuperate with a good night's rest. Work out your suitable bedtime, and then, if possible, wake up without an alarm clock. Every day you give your body the chance to wake up naturally, you will be reaffirming your natural sleep pattern.

Make your sleep space a safe place without technology. Leave the distractions of the day outside, get under some nice bed sheets, rest your head on the pillow and get your rest in.

Seven Practice Recommendations

- Go to bed at a healthy time
- Wake up without an alarm when you can
- Find your natural sleep pattern
- Avoid bright light in the evening
- Try blue-blocking glasses
- Sleep outside
- Sleep more

CONCLUSION

THANK YOU FOR taking the time to learn about the Seven Practices. You are building awareness of your well-being by reading this book.

We must continue to find a blend between the humans we used to be and the humans we want to be. We can put aside the distraction of growth and expansion into the future that has stopped us from nurturing ourselves. We can continue to show that the human species can adapt over time, and we must ensure that we are ready to make positive changes.

As much as I romanticize our wild past of hunting, foraging, and fishing as a community, I understand that this was never meant to be the pinnacle of human evolution. Or, instead, if it was the peak of human evolution, it should not be the peak of human society.

The humans we are descended from appear in records to be physically and mentally more stable and well-rounded than many of the people that make up our global society today. However, they were never the end goal for our species.

With many of us having undergone countless generations of domestication, we could likely never return to the physical state we were in during our hunter-gatherer past. However, that does not mean we cannot try to seek the same mental or spiritual well-being that these small groups of primarily nomadic humans were known to tap into.

These humans lived sustainably and developed an intimate understanding of place and purpose. Coupled with the smaller skill set needed by indigenous groups to survive, they could all become expert practitioners and teachers of what was needed to live long, happy lives—primarily the knowledge of how to safely and simply access food, water and shelter.

This focus on these skills allowed them to have a very intimate relationship with their survival, successfully operating as a species on Earth for 300,000 years. At no other point in evolution has humanity enjoyed the stability it did during those formative years as hunter-gatherers. Still, if we make the right choices and choose the right path forward, we can forge our path of stability Beyond Domestication.

For all the pros of the hunter-gatherer lifestyle, I do not believe they were supposed to be the end of our story. I refuse to believe that the approach to agriculture forged 11,000 years ago in Gobekli Tepe was a simple mistake and that everything that has come since has been a side effect of that mistake. However, there can be no doubt that we are still very much in the formative years of our societal development and that the world we have built around us will have to change considerably as we continue developing.

One day, despite all our hard work to nurture it back to health, the Earth will be gone. The sun that has fostered life on this planet we call home will not last forever, and at some point in the distant future, it will enter the second stage of its life, completely altering the location of the habitable zone in our galaxy.

Overnight temperatures on Earth will soar, causing our atmosphere to burn away, destroying all life as we know it.

Without that fateful invention of agriculture, we may never have moved past the hunter-gatherer stage of humanity, leaving us blissfully unaware of the reality of our situation; that we are hurtling through an infinite Universe, travelling millions of miles an hour, at constant risk of asteroid bombardment or the more long-term risk of the collapse of the sun.

We have come so far in 11,000 years. But as I look around at my fellow humans, I am concerned by the level of disconnect people have with the Seven Practices.

We need to once again tap into our feelings and emotions by listening to what feels good instead of following the preset road map of life laid out for us by our parents, education, TV and much more.

We are standing at a precipice where even one more small step down the path of greed could cause the future of humanity to disappear from right under our feet.

It does not take a genius to see that our planet is hurting. Around the world, natural disasters are worsening each year, and with COVID, we have seen a viral pandemic send our entire society into lockdown. What more has to happen before we can put growth aside and look inwards at ourselves, our friends, family and community?

We must nurture a deeper practice of food, water, air, sunlight, movement, mindfulness and sleep. We need to practice gratitude for existence now that, despite all the insurmountable odds, our species has been capable of finding life in this tiny spot in the Universe. And that you, as an individual, are at the end of a long chain of evolution going back to those first moments of life on Earth (and potentially even further).

What will happen if we can recognize our role in encouraging nature reconnection to continue?

What happens if we do not?

The lessons provided in this book are not the bible for human living. It is guidance and ideas for how you can rewild your well-being, reconnect to nature, and make more sustainable decisions for the planet.

Each of us is different, and in this journey to reimagine a new future, you must regularly check in with your feelings. When you regularly check in with yourself, you build awareness and ensure that each step you take improves how you feel.

As we reconnect with ourselves, our sense of place and our community, we will build the resilience to endure difficult moments. There is a world in reach that allows us to retain all the benefits of our global society, such as science and technology, without losing ourselves in the process.

The society that grows from this must find a way to improve its fundamental relationships with food, water, air and sunlight if it is ever going to recover some of the resilience that years of domestication have taken from us.

The humans that form part of this new society must do so with an active practice of movement, mindfulness, and sleep to ensure that we do not worsen the global crisis of mental health that we are all witnessing right now.

The simple fact is, to reach the future, we must be better. Only the most avid climate change deniers could confidently say that humanity's long-term future on Earth is firmly secure.

If we make it beyond this precarious time, we will do so because we have reconnected to nature. And to give nature the best chance, we must reinvent how we live, work, and play in our communities.

We must replace the tame with the wild in our lives and across the globe. As a society, we can change how we operate to give nature the best opportunity to take its true course. No one person can accomplish all this on their own. If we are to recover, this will take organized action from all around the world at all levels.

Due to our predicament, it may feel overwhelming to even think of where to begin on your rewilding journey. The key is to start small and grow from there. You will not achieve anything by going at it 110 percent and burning the candle at both ends. There must be a blend between how we live now and how we want to live. Otherwise, change cannot occur. It will take time for the world to change, and we can support it by recognizing when things are improving with gratitude and positivity.

If we can empower ourselves to make change first in our own lives, it will be possible to support our community to make changes in theirs. Only then will we have started to move Beyond Domestication.

The observations and research I have shared in this book helped me to remission from Crohn's disease. But more importantly, along the way, I found my path to a more engaged and thriving well-being supported by a healthy mind, body and soul.

I strive to live what I write by rewilding my behaviors and environment to protect myself, my friends and my family from the many risks associated with living within our society.

As I said at the beginning of this book, we live in the harshest environment we have ever faced and must take responsibility for our vision of the future. As individuals, we must feel empowered to put our health and well-being before the expectations and distractions of a domesticated society.

Only by visualizing can we begin to move forward. We can continue to heal by acknowledging what we do not know and seeking new information.

The good news is that we are on a positive path, with more research each day uncovering further understanding of both the human body and mind, but we must never let that stop us from building an awareness of how we feel.

By engaging positively with each of the Seven Practices: food, water, air, sunlight, movement, mindfulness, and sleep, you are committing to a healthier future for yourself. By focusing on what will truly make you feel better as an individual, you can build the platform to support others.

For now, the baton has passed to you.

Take the Seven Practices with you. Take this new knowledge into communities and support sustainability within your place and use it to help those closest to you with their own rewilding journey.

ACKNOWLEDGMENTS

BEYOND **D**OMESTICATION, **THE** company, started with this book in December 2019, a few months after I lost my mum to breast cancer. That loss, along with my changing view of health and well-being, led to the formation of the Seven Practices, and as the book came together, the company grew from that.

The Seven Practices were a natural step from the rewilding journey my wife Amber-Rose and I had been on since 2017. However, without a doubt, I would not be sitting here as a published author without the unwavering support that she has given me throughout my journey. Amber has supported me through all of my weird rewilding efforts, from toe shoes to cold swimming, and we have both learned so much together.

Despite Amber not being an author on this project, she has had a big hand in every step. Reading all the research, going over specific paragraphs and ultimately getting out into nature with me to rewild our lives.

To my mum, I feel you may have been the catalyst for me to take action after losing you in July 2019. I know you would be so proud to see this book on the shelves and even more proud to hear I achieved remission from Crohn's.

Dad, you are my biggest fan, and I love you for that. You are one in a million and the best parent any son could wish for. Keep windsurfing! To my sister, the genius vet, thank you for our debates. You have helped me to understand research better and strengthen my scientific arguments.

Thanks to my publisher, Hatherleigh Press, especially Andrew Flach and Ryan Tumambing. For their thoughtful and considered edits throughout, thank you to Ryan Kennedy and Hannah Renouard. From the first meeting, it was clear Hatherleigh understood the vision for the book, and I think that comes through in the final copy.

One man who has been there from the very beginning is our lead advisor, Raymond Sykes. A long-time family friend and ex-CEO, Raymond took Amber and me under his wing from the first moment, helping us to nurture Beyond Domestication into the business it is today.

Thank you to all of the initial advisory team. Under your guidance in 2021, we made some small but significant changes to the Seven Practices, shaping it into what they are today.

It is always nice to reconnect with old friends, and years after going to school together, Dr. Ed Caddye and I reconnected because of our passion for supporting people to find health and well-being in nature. Ed's knowledge of research and ability to translate that into practical guidance for his patients is a shining example of what the future of medicine can look like.

Mike Holland, thank you for openly and willingly sharing your experience, knowledge and wisdom with me over the years. Your mentoring has left a mark on me that I will try to pay forward. You have taught me so much about mindfulness, and I hope I did you justice!

I could not have asked for a better pair to guide me with the Food chapter. Heather Rosa, Dean at the Institute of Optimum Nutrition and Jeff Webster, founder of Hunter and Gather, did not hold back. Their advice gave me the confidence to follow the research and to address some underlying problems with the quality of our food rather than tip-toe around them.

Thank you to my supportive employer, the charity Directory of Social Change. You have always supported my journey to rewild well-being, and I could not ask for a better team to work with. To my colleagues Justin Martin and John Martin, thank you for giving me your time and expertise at a critical stage, as I got this book proposal ready to send to publishers.

Through my charity work with DSC, it has been a pleasure to work with many environmental charities. When I met Mike Winstanley, he was looking after conservation for the Severn River Trusts, and I instantly started badgering him to become an advisor. I can only thank him for giving up his busy time, especially during a house move, to guide Beyond Domestication and the Water chapter through its early stages.

If you want someone to take you mindfully into cold water, look no further than Breatheolution, Kevin O'Neill. I worked with Kev on the incredible Unguarded Warrior retreats, and he took my cold water virginity. His mindful approach, alongside his knowledge of breathing, was of huge support during the Water and Air chapters.

They say not to judge a book by its cover, but if I had to judge this book by its cover, I would be pretty chuffed. Thank you to Ali Al Amine for your incredible work! Thank you as well to the talented book designer Micaela Alcaino. It is nice to have talented friends, and when I met Micaela at an archery class, I never expected she would end up being such a support through the whole publishing process.

Lastly, I want to thank you, the reader. It is a beautiful experience to watch everything you have dreamed about for the last four years grow into an actual book that people can buy and read. And I do not take lightly the time you have spent reading.

Thank you for the trust.

I will keep spreading the message of the Seven Practices, and I will always be grateful to anyone who joins us on that journey.

ABOUT THE AUTHOR

GEORGE **K**NIGHT **IS** an author and rewilder. He and his wife, Amber-Rose, are the Co-Founders of Beyond Domestication, a UK-based company specializing in nature retreats and rewilding walks. They guide people to learn about the Seven Practices through foraging, airbathing, barefoot movement, wild swimming and other natural practices.

George is also a passionate trainer, connecting with individuals from various organizations across the UK and beyond.

You'll often find George with Amber-Rose on a mountain or in a forest, wild camping and swimming..

REFERENCES

Introduction

1. Symmes, P., 2010. *Turkey: Archeological Dig Reshaping Human History*. [online] Newsweek. Available at: <https://www.newsweek.com/turkey-archeological-dig-reshaping-human-history-75101>

2. Rewilding Europe. n.d. *Tauros | Rewilding Europe*. [online] Available at: <https://rewildingeurope.com/rewilding-in-action/wildlife-comeback/tauros/>

3. Theofanopoulou, C., Gastaldon, S., O'Rourke, T., Samuels, B., Martins, P., Delogu, F., Alamri, S. and Boeckx, C., 2018. Correction: Self-domestication in Homo sapiens: Insights from comparative genomics. *PLOS ONE*, 13(5), p.e0196700.

4. Stringer, C., 2014. *Why Have Our Brains Started to Shrink?*. [online] Scientific American. Available at: <https://www.scientificamerican.com/article/why-have-our-brains-started-to-shrink/>

5. Dugatkin, L. and Trut, L., 2017. How to Tame a Fox (and Build a Dog).

6. Kaiser, S., Hennessy, M. and Sachser, N., 2015. Domestication affects the structure, development and stability of biobehavioural profiles. *Frontiers in Zoology*, 12(Suppl 1), p.S19.

7. Mind.org.uk. 2020. *How common are mental health problems?*. [online] Available at: <https://www.mind.org.uk/information-

support/types-of-mental-health-problems/statistics-and-facts-about-mental-health/how-common-are-mental-health-problems/#one>

8. Bratman, G., Hamilton, J., Hahn, K., Daily, G. and Gross, J., 2015. Nature experience reduces rumination and subgenual prefrontal cortex activation. Proceedings of the National Academy of Sciences, 112(28), pp.8567-8572.

Food

9. 2014. *Soil Fertility and Erosion.* [online] Available at: <https://www.globalagriculture.org/report-topics/soil-fertility-and-erosion.html>

10. Countryside. 2019. What is soil health and why does it matter?. [online] Available at: <https://www.countrysideonline.co.uk/food-and-farming/protecting-the-environment/what-is-soil-health-and-why-does-it-matter/>

11. Swain, T., 1972. Plants in the Development of Modern Medicine. [Erscheinungsort nicht ermittelbar]: Harvard University Press.

12. Spector, T., 2017. Twin Studies. [online] Serious Science. Available at: <https://serious-science.org/twin_studies-8463>

13. Avis-Riordan, K., 2022. 8 things we've learnt about the world's plants and fungi. [online] Kew Gardens. Available at: <https://www.kew.org/read-and-watch/state-of-the-worlds-plants-and-fungi-2020-report>

14. Dunn, R., 2018. *Never Out of Season.* Back Bay Books Little BRN.

15. Koeppel, D., 2009. *Banana.* [New York]: Plume.

16. Bangun, Prajanto, Nusantoro, 2018. Food production: From farm to fork. In Preparation and Processing of Religious and Cultural Foods.

17. Jack Cincotta. 2020. *Nutritional Balance with Nose-to-Tail Eating—Jack Cincotta.* [online] Available at: <https://jackcincotta. com/2020/08/13/nutritional-balance-with-nose-to-tail-eating/>

18. Axe, J., 2020. The Collagen Diet.

19. Mckenna, M., 2018. How the 'Chicken of Tomorrow' Contest in 1948 Created the Bird We Eat Today. [online] National Geographic. Available at: <https://www.nationalgeographic.com/ environment/article/poultry-food-production-agriculture-mckenna>

20. O'Brien, C., 2017. 3-year-old child would weigh 28 stone if it grew as fast as a supermarket chicken. [online] RSPCA. Available at: <https://news.rspca.org.uk/2017/01/26/3-year-old-child-would-weigh-28-stone-if-it-grew-as-fast-as a supermarket-chicken/>

21. Wyness, L., Weichselbaum, E., O'Connor, A., Williams, E., Benelam, B., Riley, H. and Stanner, S., 2011. Red meat in the diet: an update. Nutrition Bulletin, 36(1), pp.34-77.

22. Organuary. 2022. Nutritional Benefits Of Organ Meats. [online] Available at: <https://organuary.com/nutrition/>

23. Paul, C., Leser, S. and Oesser, S., 2019. Significant Amounts of Functional Collagen Peptides Can Be Incorporated in the Diet While Maintaining Indispensable Amino Acid Balance. Nutrients, 11(5), p.1079.

24. Alcock, R., Shaw, G., Tee, N. and Burke, L., 2019. Plasma Amino Acid Concentrations After the Ingestion of Dairy and Collagen Proteins, in Healthy Active Males. Frontiers in Nutrition, 6.

25. Lenardon, M., Munro, C. and Gow, N., 2010. Chitin synthesis and fungal pathogenesis. *Current Opinion in Microbiology,* 13(4), pp.416-423.

26. Tan, S. and Tatsumura, Y., 2015. Alexander Fleming (1881–1955): Discoverer of penicillin. *Singapore Medical Journal*, 56(07), pp.366-367.

27. Power, R., Salazar-García, D., Straus, L., González Morales, M. and Henry, A., 2015. Microremains from El Mirón Cave human dental calculus suggest a mixed plant–animal subsistence economy during the Magdalenian in Northern Iberia. *Journal of Archaeological Science*, 60, pp.39-46.

28. 2018. *State of the World's Fungi.* [online] Kew Gardens. Available at: <https://stateoftheworldsfungi.org/>

29. Shao, Y. et al. 2019 'Stunted microbiota and opportunistic pathogen colonization in caesarean-section birth', Nature, 574(7776), pp. 117–121.

30. BBC News. 2018. *'World's oldest brewery' found in cave in Israel, say researchers.* [online] Available at: <https://www.bbc.co.uk/news/world-middle-east-45534133>

31. Katz, S. and Fallon Morell, S., 2016. *Wild Fermentation.* White River Junction, Vermont: Chelsea Green Publishing.

32. HAAS, L., 1998. Louis Pasteur (1822-95). Journal of Neurology, Neurosurgery & Psychiatry, 64(3), pp.330-330.

33. MacDonald, L., Brett, J., Kelton, D., Majowicz, S., Snedeker, K. and SARGEANT, J., 2011. A Systematic Review and Meta-Analysis of the Effects of Pasteurization on Milk Vitamins, and Evidence for Raw Milk Consumption and Other Health-Related Outcomes. *Journal of Food Protection*, 74(11), pp.1814-1832.

34. Spector, T., 2017. *What a hunter-gatherer diet does to the body.* [online] CNN. Available at: <https://edition.cnn.com/2017/07/05/health/hunter-gatherer-diet-tanzania-the-conversation/index.html>

35. Bosely, S., 2018. *Most common childhood cancer 'partly caused by lack of infection'*. [online] the Guardian. Available at: <https://www.theguardian.com/society/2018/may/21/most-common-childhood-cancer-partly-caused-by-lack-of-infection>

36. Marshall, M., 2019. *Why humans have evolved to drink milk*. [online] BBC. Available at: <https://www.bbc.com/future/article/20190218-when-did-humans-start-drinking-cows-milk>

37. Foodbeast. 2012. *Map of Milk Consumption & Lactose Intolerance Around the World*. [online] Available at: <https://www.foodbeast.com/news/map-of-milk-consumption-lactose-intolerance-around-the-world/>

38. Massey, L.K., Roman-Smith, H. and Sutton, R.A.L. (1993) 'Effect of dietary oxalate and calcium on urinary oxalate and risk of formation of calcium oxalate kidney stones', *Journal of the American Dietetic Association*, 93(8), pp. 901–906. doi:10.1016/0002-8223(93)91530-4.

39. Lorenz, E.C. *et al.* (2013) 'Update on oxalate Crystal Disease', *Current Rheumatology Reports*, 15(7). doi:10.1007/s11926-013-0340-4.

40. de Cabo, R. and Mattson, M., 2019. Effects of Intermittent Fasting on Health, Aging, and Disease. New England Journal of Medicine, 381(26), pp.2541-2551.

Water

41. Gill, N., 2018. Ancient Rome's Futuristic Water Systems. [online] ThoughtCo. Available at: <https://www.thoughtco.com/aqueducts-water-supply-sewers-ancient-rome-117076>

42. Dieter, C. and Maupin, M., 2015. Public supply and domestic water use in the United States, 2015 | U.S. Geological Survey. [online] U.S. Geological Survey. Available at: <https://www.usgs.gov/

publications/public-supply-and-domestic-water-use-united-
states-2015>

43. Heid, M., 2014. Does drinking old water make you sick?. [online]
     Time. Available at: <https://time.com/3104999/old-water-sick/>

44. Coldwell, W., 2021. In at the deep end: the activists plunging into
     the wild swimming campaign. [online] the Guardian. Available at:
     <https://www.theguardian.com/lifeandstyle/2021/sep/19/in-at-
     the-deep-end-the-activists-plunging-into-the-wild-swimming-
     campaign>

45. Lindquist, J. and Mertens, P., 2018. Cold shock proteins: from
     cellular mechanisms to pathophysiology and disease. Cell
     Communication and Signaling, 16(1).

46. Smedley, T., 2017. Is the world running out of fresh water?.
     [online] Bbc.com. Available at: <https://www.bbc.com/future/
     article/20170412-is-the-world-running-out-of-fresh-water>

47. Souza, C., Kirchhoff, F., Oliveira, B., Ribeiro, J. and Sales, M.,
     2019. Long-Term Annual Surface Water Change in the Brazilian
     Amazon Biome: Potential Links with Deforestation, Infrastructure
     Development and Climate Change. Water, 11(3), p.566.

48. Wildmadagascar.org. n.d. Erosion in Madagascar. [online]
     Available at: <https://www.wildmadagascar.org/conservation/
     erosion.html>

49. Hov, Ø., Cubasch, U. and Fischer, E., 2013. Extreme weather events
     in Europe. Oslo: Norwegian Meteorological Institute.

50. Cassidy, E., 2018. 5 Major Cities Threatened by Climate Change
     and Sea Level Rise |. [online] TheCityFix. Available at: <https://
     thecityfix.com/blog/5-major-cities-threatened-climate-change-
     sea-level-rise-emily-cassidy/>

51. Kulp, S. and Strauss, B., 2019. New elevation data triple estimates of global vulnerability to sea-level rise and coastal flooding. Nature Communications, 10(1).

52. McGrath, M., 2019. Climate change: Warming to drive 'robust increase' in UK flooding. [online] BBC News. Available at: <https://www.bbc.co.uk/news/science-environment-49731591>

53. Flyn, C., 2018. 'People think the deer are lovely. Then they learn more about it': the deer cull dilemma. [online] the Guardian. Available at: <https://www.theguardian.com/news/2018/feb/20/deer-cull-dilemma-scottish-highlands>

54. Barnett, B., 2019. Beavers released in Cropton Forest as pioneering UK trial gets underway. [online] Yorkshirepost.co.uk. Available at: <https://www.yorkshirepost.co.uk/news/environment/beavers-released-cropton-forest-pioneering-uk-trial-gets-underway-1756554>

55. Newton, G., 2020. Beavers introduced to Yorkshire in 2019 may have prevented Storm Dennis flooding with their dams. [online] Yorkshirepost.co.uk. Available at: <https://www.yorkshirepost.co.uk/news/environment/beavers-introduced-yorkshire-2019-may-have-prevented-storm-dennis-flooding-their-dams-1889853>

Air

56. Black, R., 2010. The History of Air. [online] Smithsonian Magazine. Available at: <https://www.smithsonianmag.com/science-nature/the-history-of-air-21082166/>

57. Beelen, R., Raaschou-Nielsen, O., Stafoggia, M., Andersen, Z., Weinmayr, G. and Hoffmann, B., 2014. Air pollution and human health: Long-term exposure to fine particulate air pollution associated with natural-cause mortality. Clean Air Journal, 24(1), p.6.

58. Poslusny, C., 2018. Off-gassing and Outgassing: What's the Difference and Where Is It from?. [online] Molekule.science. Available at: <https://molekule.science/off-gassing-and-outgassing-whats-the-difference-and-where-is-it-from/>

59. Golde, K., 2022. New Mattress Smell & Off-Gassing Guide | Mattress Clarity. [online] Mattress Clarity. Available at: <https://www.mattressclarity.com/blog/new-mattress-smell-mattress-off-gassing/>

60. Thompson, D., 2019. Is Your Mattress Releasing Toxins While You Sleep?. [online] WebMD. Available at: <https://www.webmd.com/sleep-disorders/news/20190710/is-your-mattress-releasing-toxins-while-you-sleep#2>

61. CustomMade. 2015. How Scared Should You Be of Off-Gassing?. [online] Available at: <https://www.custommade.com/blog/off-gassing/>

62. Wolverton, B., Johnson, A. and Bounds, K., 1989. Interior Landscape Plants for Indoor Air Pollution Abatement.

63. Avol, E.L. *et al.* (2001) 'Respiratory effects of relocating to areas of differing air pollution levels', *American Journal of Respiratory and Critical Care Medicine*, 164(11), pp. 2067–2072. doi:10.1164/ajrccm.164.11.2102005.

64. Sinharay, R. *et al.* (2018) 'Respiratory and cardiovascular responses to walking down a traffic-polluted road compared with walking in a traffic-free area in participants aged 60 years and older with chronic lung or heart disease and age-matched healthy controls: A randomised, crossover study', *The Lancet*, 391(10118), pp. 339–349. doi:10.1016/s0140-6736(17)32643-0.

65. Lyu, B., Zeng, C., Xie, S., Li, D., Lin, W., Li, N., Jiang, M., Liu, S. and Chen, Q., 2019. Benefits of A Three-Day Bamboo Forest Therapy Session on the Psychophysiology and Immune System

Responses of Male College Students. International Journal of Environmental Research and Public Health, 16(24), p.4991.

66. Lee, J., Tsunetsugu, Y., Takayama, N., Park, B., Li, Q., Song, C., Komatsu, M., Ikei, H., Tyrväinen, L., Kagawa, T. and Miyazaki, Y., 2014. Influence of Forest Therapy on Cardiovascular Relaxation in Young Adults. Evidence-Based Complementary and Alternative Medicine, 2014, pp.1-7.

67. Zaccaro, A., Piarulli, A., Laurino, M., Garbella, E., Menicucci, D., Neri, B. and Gemignani, A., 2018. How Breath-Control Can Change Your Life: A Systematic Review on Psycho-Physiological Correlates of Slow Breathing. Frontiers in Human Neuroscience, 12.

68. McClernon, F., Westman, E. and Rose, J., 2004. The effects of controlled deep breathing on smoking withdrawal symptoms in dependent smokers. Addictive Behaviors, 29(4), pp.765-772.

69. Sciencedaily.com. 2011. Research on 'Iceman' Wim Hof suggests it may be possible to influence autonomic nervous system and immune response. [online] Available at: <https://www.sciencedaily.com/releases/2011/04/110422090203.htm>

70. Kox, M., van Eijk, L., Zwaag, J., van den Wildenberg, J., Sweep, F., van der Hoeven, J. and Pickkers, P., 2014. Voluntary activation of the sympathetic nervous system and attenuation of the innate immune response in humans. Proceedings of the National Academy of Sciences, 111(20), pp.7379-7384.

Sunlight

71. *Overview - Rickets and osteomalacia* (no date) *NHS choices.* Available at: https://www.nhs.uk/conditions/rickets-and-osteomalacia/

72. Jablonski, N., 2013. Skin: A Natural History. Berkeley, Calif: Univ. of California Press.

73. Sima, E., 2016. Sun protection and dark skin: what you need to know. [online] SBS.com. Available at: <https://www.sbs.com.au/topics/science/humans/article/2016/12/16/sun-protection-and-dark-skin-what-you-need-know>

74. Harris, S., 2006. Vitamin D and African Americans. The Journal of Nutrition, 136(4), pp.1126-1129.

75. Murray, F., 2013. Sunshine and Vitamin D. North Bergen, NJ: Basic Health Publications.

76. Klepeis, N., Nelson, W., Ott, W., Robinson, J., Tsang, A., Switzer, P., Behar, J., Hern, S. and Engelmann, W., 2001. The National Human Activity Pattern Survey (NHAPS): a resource for assessing exposure to environmental pollutants. Journal of Exposure Science & Environmental Epidemiology, 11(3), pp.231-252.

77. Chia, E., 2021. Myopia rising among kids in S'pore as screen time goes up during the pandemic. [online] The Straits Times. Available at: <https://www.straitstimes.com/life/myopia-rising-among-kids-here-as-screen-time-goes-up-during-the-pandemic>

78. Duffy, J. and Czeisler, C., 2009. Effect of Light on Human Circadian Physiology. Sleep Medicine Clinics, 4(2), pp.165-177.

79. Fricke, T., Jong, M., Naidoo, K., Sankaridurg, P., Naduvilath, T., Ho, S., Wong, T. and Resnikoff, S., 2018. Global prevalence of visual impairment associated with myopic macular degeneration and temporal trends from 2000 through 2050: systematic review, meta-analysis and modelling. British Journal of Ophthalmology, 102(7), pp.855-862.

80. Bei Yi, S., 2015. New way to look after children's eyes. [online] The Straits Times. Available at: <https://www.straitstimes.com/singapore/new-way-to-look-after-childrens-eyes>

81. Nunez, C., 2019. What Is Global Warming?. [online] National Geographic. Available at: <https://www.nationalgeographic.com/environment/article/global-warming-overview>

82. Zhao, Y. *et al.* (2018) 'Stable iridium dinuclear heterogeneous catalysts supported on metal-oxide substrate for solar water oxidation', *Proceedings of the National Academy of Sciences*, 115(12), pp. 2902–2907. doi:10.1073/pnas.1722137115.

Movement

83. Blair SN, 2009. Physical inactivity: the biggest public health problem of the 21st century. British Journal of Sports Medicine, 43:1-2

84. Levine, J., Eberhardt, N. and Jensen, M., 1999. Role of Nonexercise Activity Thermogenesis in Resistance to Fat Gain in Humans. Science, 283(5399), pp.212-214.

85. Hagger-Johnson, G., Gow, A., Burley, V., Greenwood, D. and Cade, J., 2016. Sitting Time, Fidgeting, and All-Cause Mortality in the UK Women's Cohort Study. American Journal of Preventive Medicine, 50(2), pp.154-160.

86. Mohiyeddini, C. and Semple, S., 2012. Displacement behaviour regulates the experience of stress in men. Stress, 16(2), pp.163-171.

87. Sapolsky, R., 2004. Why Zebras Don't Get Ulcers. New York: Henry Holt and Co.

88. 2013. Educating the Student Body.

89. Fritz, J., 2017. Physical Activity During Growth. Effects on Bone, Muscle, Fracture Risk and Academic Performance. Lund University: Faculty of Medicine.

90. Chevalier, G., Sinatra, S., Oschman, J. and Delany, R., 2013. Earthing (Grounding) the Human Body Reduces Blood Viscosity—a Major Factor in Cardiovascular Disease. The Journal of Alternative and Complementary Medicine, 19(2), pp.102-110.

91. Wainwright, M., 2005. Emails 'pose threat to IQ'. [online] the Guardian. Available at: <https://www.theguardian.com/technology/2005/apr/22/money.workandcareers>

92. Griffey, H., 2018. The lost art of concentration: being distracted in a digital world. [online] The Guardian. Available at: <https://www.theguardian.com/lifeandstyle/2018/oct/14/the-lost-art-of-concentration-being-distracted-in-a-digital-world>

93. Stone, L., 2009. Beyond Simple Multi-Tasking: Continuous Partial Attention. [online] Available at: <https://lindastone.net/faq/continuous-partial-attention/>

94. Curtis, A., 2011. Five Years After Banning Outdoor Ads, Brazil's Largest City Is More Vibrant Than Ever. [online] New Dream. Available at: <https://newdream.org/blog/sao-paolo-ad-ban>

Mindfulness

95. Mark, G., Gonzalez, V. and Harris, J., 2005. No task left behind?. Proceedings of the SIGCHI Conference on Human Factors in Computing Systems,.

96. Knowles, S., 2018. Mindful Eating for Weight Loss. [online] NC Cooperative Extension. Available at: <https://sampson.ces.ncsu.edu/2018/04/mindful-eating-for-weight-loss/>

97. Gelles, D., 2016. Mindful work. Boston: Mariner Books.

Sleep

98. Pacheco, D. and Rehman, A. (2023) *Chronotypes: Definition, types, & effect on sleep, Sleep Foundation*. Available at: https://www.sleepfoundation.org/how-sleep-works/chronotypes

99. Stevens, R. and Zhu, Y., 2015. Electric light, particularly at night, disrupts human circadian rhythmicity: is that a problem?.

Philosophical Transactions of the Royal Society B: Biological Sciences, 370(1667), p.20140120.

100. Davis, S., Mirick, D. and Stevens, R., 2001. Night Shift Work, Light at Night, and Risk of Breast Cancer. JNCI Journal of the National Cancer Institute, 93(20), pp.1557-1562.

101. Van Dycke, K., Rodenburg, W., van Oostrom, C., van Kerkhof, L., Pennings, J., Roenneberg, T., van Steeg, H. and van der Horst, G., 2015. Chronically Alternating Light Cycles Increase Breast Cancer Risk in Mice. Current Biology, 25(14), pp.1932-1937.

102. Low Blue Lights. 2022. What LBL Does. [online] Available at: <https://lowbluelights.com/what-lbl-does/>

103. Coren, S., 1996. Daylight Savings Time and Traffic Accidents. New England Journal of Medicine, 334(14), pp.924-925.

104. Janszky, I. and Ljung, R., 2008. Shifts to and from Daylight Saving Time and Incidence of Myocardial Infarction. New England Journal of Medicine, 359(18), pp.1966-1968.

105. Liu, C., Politch, J., Cullerton, E., Go, K., Pang, S. and Kuohung, W., 2017. Impact of daylight savings time on spontaneous pregnancy loss in in vitro fertilization patients. Chronobiology International, 34(5), pp.571-577.

106. Berk, M., Dodd, S., Hallam, K., Berk, L., Gleeson, J. and Henry, M., 2008. Small shifts in diurnal rhythms are associated with an increase in suicide: The effect of daylight saving. Sleep and Biological Rhythms, 6(1), pp.22-25.

107. Hayashi, M., Motoyoshi, N. and Hori, T., 2005. Recuperative Power of a Short Daytime Nap With or Without Stage 2 Sleep. Sleep,.

108. Jacoby, J. (2018) *The undeferred dreams of Elias Howe and Madame C. J. Walker - The Boston Globe, BostonGlobe.com.* Available at: https://www.bostonglobe.com/opinion/2018/

03/23/the-undeferred-dreams-elias-howe-and-madame-walker/
GA3ajqwnq4UiVoFe3HQERP/story.html

109. Payne, J. and Kensinger, E., 2010. Sleep's Role in the Consolida-
tion of Emotional Episodic Memories. Current Directions in
Psychological Science, 19(5), pp.290-295.

110. Cajochen, C., Altanay-Ekici, S., Münch, M., Frey, S., Knoblauch,
V. and Wirz-Justice, A., 2013. Evidence that the Lunar Cycle
Influences Human Sleep. Current Biology, 23(15), pp.1485-1488.